HEALING WITHIN:

The Complete Guide to Colon Health

Written and Compiled by
Stanley Weinberger, C.M.T.

© 1988, 1996 by Stanley Weinberger
Healing Within Products
P.O. Box 1013
Larkspur, CA 94977-1013
Telephone: (415) 454-6677
Fax only: (415) 454-6659
E-mail: healing@nbn.com

1st Edition 1988
2nd Edition, 1993
3rd Edition, 1st Printing 1996

HEALING WITHIN: The Complete Guide to Colon Health
can be purchased at most health food stores and bookstores.
For mail orders, see order forms on pages 291-297.

Edited by Beth Kuper
Typography by Allen M. Crider
Proofreading by Margaret Dodd

ISBN 0-9616184-7-7

Printed in the U.S.A.

Note to the Reader

HEALING WITHIN: The Complete Guide to Colon Health does not claim to substitute for a physician's care, nor does it advocate specific solutions to individual problems. The physicians and experts providing the enclosed information have substantiated their claims as well as is possible considering that data on health and nutrition are subject to change as we learn more.

Before following the self-help advice given in this book, readers are earnestly urged to give careful consideration to the nature of their particular health problem and to consult a competent physician if they are in any doubt.

This book should not be regarded as a substitute for professional medical treatment. Every care has been taken to ensure accuracy of the content. Still, the author and publisher cannot accept legal responsibility for any problem arising out of the methods described in this book.

Dedication

Dedicated to the memory of Evelyn Wanek,
for all the many years of devoted service
she gave to colon therapy.
Bless you.

Contents

List of Illustrations xii
About the Author xiii
Introduction xiv

CHAPTER 1
Your Colon Needs Attention! 1
Colon Health 3
   The Amazing Digestive System 6
   The Length of the Human Digestive Tract
   Compared To the Human Form 7
   Colon Therapy Chart 8
   History of Colon Therapy 9
   Do You Fit This Description? 10
   Toxic Buildup 10
   Imbalances of the Colon 11
   Normal and Abnormal Colons 12-13
   Attitudes that Promote Intestinal Inefficiency 14
   Causes of Constipation 14
   Constipating Foods and Drinks 15
   Attitudes that Promote Health 16
   Colon Reflex Chart 18

CHAPTER 2
Suggestions To Improve Bowel Function 19
   Liquids To Improve Bowel Function 22
   Food Combining and Amounts 22
   Foods To Avoid or Replace 23
   Cooking Suggestions 23
   Bowel Function 24
   Exercise and Meditation 24
Slant-Board Exercises 25
   Directions for Using the Slant Board 26
   Slant-Board Exercise Positions 27-30
The Ileocecal Valve Syndrome, by Dr. David G. Williams 31
   What and Where Is This Valve? 31
   When the Valve Sticks Shut 32
   When the Valve Sticks Open 32

CONTENTS

Why Me? 32
Open Ileocecal Valve—What to Do 33
Stopping the Flu Dead in Its Tracks 33
Ileocecal Valve Reflex Points 35

CHAPTER 3
Colon Therapy: Pathway to Vibrant Health 37
Benefits of Colon Therapy 39
Six Colon X-Rays 41
Colon Therapy with Oxygen 42
Colon-Cleansing Procedure 43
Commonly Asked Questions about Colon Therapy 44

CHAPTER 4
Healing Within Four- or Seven-Day Colon Cleansing Program . 49
Instructions 52
Products and Procedures 53
Apple Cider Vinegar Drink 53
Castor Oil Packs for the Immune System 53
Colon 8 Intestinal Cleanser 54
DDS Acidophilus Culture 54
Dr. Jensen's Broth 55
Dry Skin Brushing 55
Fresh Vegetable Juices 56
KB-11 Tablets 56
Pau D'Arco Tea 57
Whole Life Food Blend 57
Four-Day Colon Cleansing Program 59
Seven-Day Colon Cleansing Program 59
Suggested Time Schedule 60
Products Needed for the Colon Cleansing Program 61
Ending Your Colon Cleansing Program 62
Food Time 63

CHAPTER 5
Lactobacillus Acidophilus: The Well-Kept Secret 65
Lactobacillus Acidophilus: The Friendly Bacteria 67
Lactobacillus Acidophilus History, by Keith W. Sehnert, M.D. . . 68
Lactobacillus Uses 69

Not All Lactobicilli Are the Same 69
Therapeutic Effects of DDS 70
Nutritional Effects 70
Miscellaneous Actions 70
Comparison of Commercial Products 71
  General Summary of DDS Advantages 71
  Conclusions 73
*Our Internal Microbial Community—Maintaining
  the Healthy Balance* 75
  Three Phase Intestinal Flora Rebuilding Program 77

CHAPTER 6
Candida Albicans: The Quiet Epidemic 79
Candida Albicans Overgrowth, by William Wolcott 81
  What is Candida? 81
  How Do You Get Candida? 82
  Do You Have Candida? 82
  Causes of Candida Overgrowth 83
  What Are the Signs of Candida Infections? 86
  How Do You Know You Have Candida? 87
  How Do You Reduce Candida Overgrowth? 89
  Proper Diet 90
  Conclusion 92
How to Fight Candida and Survive, by Tom Valentine 93
  A Natural War 94
  AIDS-Plus 94
  Candida Albicans 96
  Contributing Factors 100
Candida Albicans Self-Test 101
  Introduction 101
  Instructions 101
  Section A: History 102
  Section B: Major Symptoms 104
  Section C: Other Symptoms 106
  Scoring 108
Oxygen Therapy 109
  Why It Should Be of Interest to Everyone 109
  Summary 110
Ozone: Its Therapeutic Action 113

CHAPTER 7
Products for Candida Control 117
OXY-OXC 119
 The Next Generation in Superoxygenation 119
 What Are the Contents of OXY-OXC? 121
 What Does OXY-OXC Do? 121
 Why Is OXY-OXC Needed? 121
 How Does OXY-OXC Work? 121
 How is OXY-OXC Made? 122
Pau D'Arco Tea and Colon 8 Intestinal Cleanser 123
 Colon 8 Intestinal Cleanser 123
DDS Acidophilus Culture 124
 Not All Lactobacilli Are the Same 124
 Therapeutic Effects of DDS 124
 Nutritional Effects 125
Caprystatin, Kaprycidin-A & Orithrush-D 126
Latero Flora 127
Travacid X (HCl), by Tom Valentine 129
 A Better Stimulant 130
 Healthy Lymph 131
Coenzyme Q10 134
 Benefits 135
Immuno-Quest 136
Natur-Earth 139
 An Amazing New Breakthrough in
  Immune Stimulation and Healing 139
 SBOs in the Human Diet 139
 The Making of Natur-Earth 140
 Secret Process 142
 Dramatic Healing Results! 142
 How It Works: A Basic Outline 143
 Natur-Earth and the Human Immune System:
  The Inside Details 145
 Summary of Natur-Earth's Unique Immune-Stimulating Actions 154
 More Amazing Therapeutic Benefits 155
 Stimulates Cellular Self-Repair 155
 Provides Powerful Anti-Oxidants 156
 Corrects Nutrient Absorption Deficiencies 157

A Major New Weapon against Viruses, Candida, Allergies,
by Dr. Robert W. Bradford *161*
   Universal Reactive Syndrome *162*
   The Breakthrough of Dioxychlor *164*
   The Background *165*
   Other Cytotoxic Oxidizing Agents Used Clinically *167*
   Cytoxicity of Dioxychlor *168*
Quote from Leon Chaitow, N.D., D.O. *169*

CHAPTER 8
Eight-Week Candida Overgrowth Elimination Program *171*
Required Products *173*
   Candida Die-Off Reactions *174*
   Colon Therapy Recommendation *174*
   Colonic . . . A Gentle Irrigation for Your Colon *174*
   Dietary Instructions *176*
Schedule and Dosage *178*
Post-Program Maintenance *181*
Letters from Satisfied Clients *183*

CHAPTER 9
Parasites: An Epidemic in Disguise *189*
   The Far Side, Carton by Gary Larson *190*
Worms Outrank Cancer as Man's Deadliest Enemy,
   by Dolly Katz *197*
Parasites More Common than Believed, Study Says,
   by Ronald Kotulak *199*
Parasites and AIDS, by Rev. Hanna Kroeger *202*
The Protozoal Syndrome, by Louis Parrish, M.D. *204*
   A Brief History *204*
   Millions Affected in U. S. A. Alone *205*
   Effects on the Immune System *205*
   Alarming Misconceptions *206*
   Symptoms *207*
   Proper Diagnostic Use of the Rectal Swab Technique (RST) . . . *208*
   Treatment *209*
   Medicines Available *209*
   Counseling Patients on Prevention *210*
   Conclusions *211*

CONTENTS

A Brief Update of the Current Global Parasitic Epidemic 212
  A Perspective of Modern Anti-Pathogenic
    Therapeutic Modalities 212
  Parasitic Disease Incidences Worldwide 213
  Parasite Questionnaire 214
Laboratory Description of Common Parasites 215
  Common Parasitic Diseases 218

CHAPTER 10
A New Generation of Herbal Parasite Fighters Has Arrived! ... 219
Presenting . . . The Healing Within
  Parasite Elimination Program 221
    The Colon Complements 221
    Some of the Organisms Affected by Gozarte, Udarte,
      Neo-Pararte, Pasaloc, and Padapco 222
    Gozarte 223
    Neo-Pararte 224
    Udarte 225
    Pasaloc 226
    Padapco 227
    Recommendations 228
    K-Min 228
    Black Walnut Tincture 229
    Castor Oil Capsules 229
    Healing Within Intestinal Cleanser 230
    Latero Flora 231
    Immune System Strengtheners 232
    Echinacea 232
    Shitake Mushroom Capsules 233
    Acidophilus 233
    Post-Program Maintenance 234
    Intestinalis Herbal Cleanser 234
  Letters from Satisfied Clients 235
  Healing Within Parasite Elimination Kits 242

CHAPTER 11
Metabolic Typing: The Commonsense
  Guide to Proper Nutrition 247
    Creating Clarity from Confusion 250

The HEALTHEXCEL System 251
Metabolic Typing: Understanding Body Language 254
Information About HEALTHEXCEL 256

CHAPTER 12
Articles by Other Authors 259
High-Colonic Irrigation, by Carol Signorella 261
Colonic Irrigation, by Angela Bell 267
Psychology of the Colon, by John Harvey Kellogg, M.D. 271
Colon Therapy: The Natural Way to Renewed
  Health, by Sheila Shea 274
    The Colon Is a Neighbor 275

CHAPTER 13
Quotes From America's Leading Experts on Colon Health 283
Quotes from Bernard Jensen, D.C., Ph.D. 285
    Bernard Jensen, D.C., Ph.D. 286
Quotes from Norman Walker, D.Sc. 287
    Norman W. Walker, D.Sc. 288
References and Suggested Reading 289

ORDER FORMS 291
    Healing Within Products Price List 292
    Shipping and Product Information 298
    Healing Within Products Order Form 300

List of Illustrations

The Amazing Digestive System 6
The Length of the Human Digestive Tract
Compared to the Human Form 7
Colon Therapy Chart 8
Normal and Abnormal Colons 12-13
Colon Reflex Chart 17
Slant-Board Exercise Positions 27-30
Ileocecal Valve Reflex Points 35
Six Colon X-Rays 41
The Far Side, Cartoon by Gary Larson 190
Common Parasitic Diseases 218
Bernard Jensen, D.C., Ph.D. 286
Norman W. Walker, D.Sc.. 288

About the Author

by Stanley Weinberger

Although I have been active in the health field for the past 20 years, my initial interest in health and finding ways to improve it was brought about by a severe decline in my own general state of health. I did not have a diagnosed disease, but still I was plagued with severe constipation, chronic back pain, excessive weight, constant fatigue, and irritability. I felt I was losing my zest for life and I was only in my mid-thirties.

After trying many different methods of treatment without showing improvement, I discovered colon therapy. Within six months and after approximately 30 treatments I had lost 70 pounds and began to regain my energy. The constipation improved and the nagging back pain all but disappeared. My outlook changed dramatically. I finally found a way to maintain and even improve my health.

Since that time, I have studied iridology (analyzing the iris of the eye for indication of bodily health and disease) with Dr. Bernard Jensen, and have studied metabolic nutrition with Dr. William Kelley and HEALTHEXCEL.

Currently, I am a Certified Metabolic Technician working with HEALTHEXCEL metabolic nutritional programs, iridology, and colon therapy. In 1988, I established the Colon Health Center in Marin County, ten miles north of San Francisco.

I want to acknowledge my editor, Beth Kuper. Without her this book would not have been possible. As an editor of numerous other books and long-time advocate of holistic health, she was a natural choice to edit *HEALING WITHIN: The Complete Guide to Colon Health.*

Writing this book was inspired by my own health experiences and the desire to make information about the wonderful benefits of colon therapy and other valuable alternative health practices more available to the general public.

Men occasionally stumble over the truth, but most pick themselves up and hurry off as if nothing had happened.
—Winston Churchill

Introduction

My purpose in writing this book is to familiarize you with a method of colon cleansing known as colonic irrigation, or colonics. This book also brings together the most current and relevant information from the works of some of the foremost authorities in the field of preventive medicine.

This new and revised edition of *HEALING WITHIN: The Complete Guide to Colon Health* includes programs for parasite elimination and candida reduction, as well as an excellent inner-cleansing program and the very latest in nutritional support and metabolic-typing programs to assist you in strengthening your immune system.

Most of us recognize the importance of bringing our automobiles in for periodic tune-ups and maintenance. We all realize that unless we take proper care of the engine, carbon deposits and other buildup can reduce its efficiency and shorten its useful life. Yet we often go on for years, sometimes even for our whole lives, without giving a thought to the importance of inner cleansing of the most miraculous machine of all: our own bodies. But when you stop and think about it, nothing makes more sense.

A simple cleansing program is the first and most important positive step you can take to establish and maintain the highest possible level of health and vitality. Throughout your life, you are exposed to many varieties of air and water pollution, pesticides in food, and toxic chemicals in the environment. These, along with improper nutrition, stress, lack of exercise, and long-term use of prescription drugs can result in the loss of vitality, weakening of the immune system, sluggish elimination and, eventually, illness. The buildup of toxins in the colon has an adverse effect on the whole body. This deterioration often takes place so slowly you may not even notice it; but nonetheless, it happens to everyone.

Colon cleansing is an effective, time-proven adjunct to any health or weight-loss program. This gentle method of cleansing and exercising the colon (large intestine) with warm water and herbs helps restore proper function and well-being to a very overworked and often toxic organ.

As you take more responsibility for your health habits, you learn to make decisions regarding your lifestyle that promote health, rather than hinder it. You contact a part of yourself that intuitively knows what is right for your emotional, physical, and spiritual health. You begin to release your fears.

You have the knowledge to heal yourself. All you have to do is begin to take charge of your body. Hopefully, this book will be an inspiration and guide to you in your quest for vibrant health.

San Anselmo, California
April 1996

Colon therapy is not intended to be a cure-all, but is a valuable procedure for a wide variety of conditions of ill health. Intestinal malfunctions are precursors of many illnesses. The restoration of intestinal elimination, too often ignored, is an important preliminary course to the restoration of health. An inefficient colon is not always the cause of sickness, but it is believed to accentuate and prolong any and all diseased conditions of the human body.

—Dr. J. E. G. Waddington

1

Your Colon Needs Attention!

The colon is the most neglected and forgotten part of the body. Colon health emphasizes prevention rather than cure. It is the most important step in maintaining or regaining vital health.

-Norman W. Walker, D.Sc.

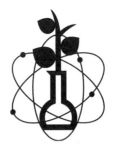

Colon Health

Your body is the house in which you live. By analogy, it is similar to the building in which you make your home. Your home needs, at the very least, periodic attention. Otherwise, the roof may leak, the plumbing may clog up, termites may drill through the floors and walls, and other innumerable signs of deterioration may make their appearance. Such is the case with your body. Every function and activity of your system, day and night, physical, mental, and emotional, is dependent upon the attention you give it.

The kind and quality of food you put into your body is of vital importance to every phase of your existence. Good nutrition regenerates the cells and tissues. It also enhances the processes by which waste matter, the undigested food, is eliminated from your body to prevent toxicity in the form of fermentation and putrefaction. This toxicity, if retained and allowed to accumulate in the body, prevents the possibility of attaining any degree of vibrant health.

The colon, a hollow tube-like organ also called the large intestine, extends from the cecum, where the small intestine empties, and continues approximately five to five-and-a-half feet down to the rectum.

The inner lining of the colon is equipped with sensitive nerves and glands. These glands aid the final stages of digestion and assimilation of food—especially minerals and water—

and help to eliminate wastes from the system. Infrequent bowel movements or periods of constipation can result in only partial decomposition of these waste substances that encrust the colon. This further hinders elimination, causing a toxic buildup in the body.

Colon therapists and researchers in degenerative diseases have shown that much of the body weight can be just waste accumulated within the 60,000 miles of blood vessels, the lymphatic system, bone joints, and intra- and extracellular regions. The largest amount of waste is found in the impactions within the colon structures: up to 50 pounds of fecal waste can accumulate over the decades.

Some of this partially digested cooked food in the small intestine and colon passes into the bloodstream and is deposited as waste throughout the system. If these wastes are calories, they can show up as obesity; excess minerals show up as arthritis; excess protein is built into cancer; fat leads to high cholesterol; and sugar leads to diabetes.

In addition, the blood eliminates many of its wastes through the walls of the colon. When these wastes from the blood arrive at the inner walls of the colon, they are unable to pass through this area if it is crammed with hardened feces. So these wastes are reabsorbed and distributed throughout the body, poisoning the blood, weakening the immune system, and causing a variety of diseases.

Wastes, along with toxins resulting from the fermentation and putrefaction of undigested food, prevent muscular contractions (known as peristaltic waves) from sweeping the packed and hardened fecal matter along the digestive canal. The result of this condition is called intestinal stasis, or constipation.

When a person is constipated, the walls of the colon are packed with accumulated feces from many months or years of intestinal cramming. The colon might be compared to a water pipe that is partly obstructed by mineral deposits and corrosion. Thus, you can imagine how proper absorption of minerals into the bloodstream and elimination of feces would not occur in a congested and impacted colon. J. H. Tilden, M.D., said:

> Without poisoning there can be no disease. In acute diseases we behold nature making her most profound effort to get rid of poison.

Relief of this situation is not a simple matter of washing out loose material lying free inside the lower third of the colon. If this were the case, enemas would be sufficient for its removal.

Colonic irrigation, however, enables the impacted fecal matter to break down and be eliminated, along with particles of old mucous from the entire length of the colon. In some cases of cleansing, one or more forms of parasites, including tapeworms, may also be eliminated. Norman W. Walker, D.Sc., wrote:

> The elimination of waste matter from the body should be meticulously taken care of by means of . . . colon irrigation whenever there is the slightest indication that the eliminative organs are becoming sluggish. In this eliminative washing out process, do not be misled into the thought that [colon cleansings] are not beneficial. Also disregard any claims that they cause loss of intestinal flora, as this is not true. No intestinal flora can exist or flourish when the fecal matter clogs up the glands in the colon that cause the flora to flourish.

The very important intestinal bacteria (friendly flora) are damaged, weakened or destroyed by antibiotics, hormones, birth control pills, and steroids. By having colon cleansings and by orally taking a strong strain of acidophilus, you have the opportunity to rebuild the friendly bacterial level that may have been disrupted or destroyed by antibiotics, whether taken years ago or recently.

Unfortunately, no long-term side effect testing has ever been done on antibiotics, so the long-term side effects of these drugs are just beginning to emerge and be recognized. One of the side effects results in a yeast overgrowth (candida) in the colon that causes multiple health problems (see Chapter 6).

The Amazing Digestive System

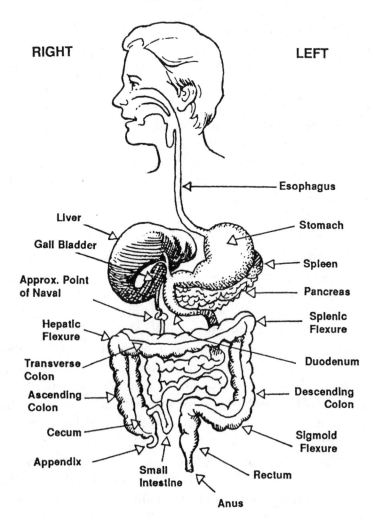

RIGHT   LEFT

Esophagus

Liver

Stomach

Gall Bladder

Spleen

Approx. Point
of Naval

Pancreas

Hepatic
Flexure

Splenic
Flexure

Transverse
Colon

Duodenum

Ascending
Colon

Descending
Colon

Cecum

Sigmoid
Flexure

Appendix

Small
Intestine

Rectum

Anus

The Length of the Human Digestive Tract Compared to the Human Form

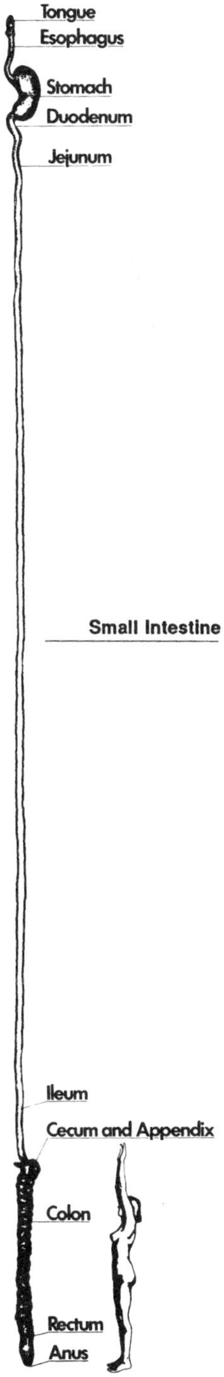

Tongue
Esophagus

Stomach
Duodenum

Jejunum

Small Intestine

Ileum

Cecum and Appendix

Colon

Rectum

Anus

(Note that the length of the digestive tract is approximately six times longer than the human form.)

Each sack in your colon, found on the colon chart, is related to another part of your body. That is why colon cleansing helps different people in so many different ways.
—Norman W. Walker, D.Sc.

Colon Therapy Chart

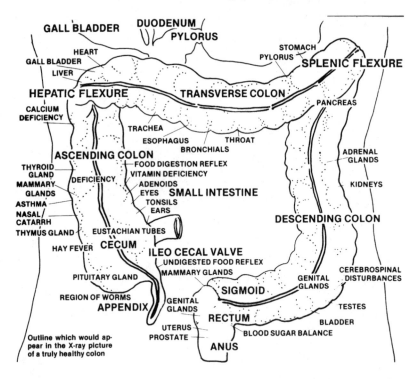

Colon therapy is recognized as an important step in maintaining or regaining health. The above chart illustrates how health and sickness have their roots in the colon. It is easy to see how an improper diet affects your colon and, in turn, inflicts pain or discomfort on the other parts of the body. Pocketing and buildup of fecal matter in various areas of the colon can affect those areas of the body indicated in the chart.

History of Colon Therapy

Despite treatment dating back to Biblical times, there still seems to be a great deal of ignorance about the healing benefits of colon therapy.

—Dr. J. E. G. Waddington

Colon therapy is a very ancient method of treatment and form of healing. Enemas were recorded as early as 1,500 B.C. in the "Ebers Papyrus," an ancient Egyptian medical document. Hippocrates, Galen, and Pare also promoted the use of enema therapy. In these earlier times, people performed an enema in a lake or river using a hollow reed to allow water to flow into the rectum. Bernard Jensen, D.C., said:

In times past, knowledge of the bowel was more widespread and people were taught how to care for the bowel. Somehow, bowel wisdom got lost and it became something that no one wanted to talk about anymore.

Enemas were at one time a more common procedure than today. Before the departure of the Lewis and Clarke expedition, a physician instructed them in the appropriateness of using enemas in cases of fever and illness. Our grandparents and great-grandparents grew up with the use of enemas as a widely accepted procedure for reversing the onset of illness. The general public's awareness and practice of this valuable health tool has diminished greatly in the past 50 years. This is due to a deliberate attempt by the American Medical Association and the orthodox medical community to withhold vital information on the benefits of colon therapy, as well as many other preventive health practices.

With the development of sophisticated colonic irrigation machines and the increasing desire among many people to return to more natural methods of dealing with their health, colon therapy once again is experiencing a return to popularity. It is estimated that there may be as many as 2,000 therapists actively practicing colon therapy in the United States.

Do You Fit This Description?

Have you ever said, "I'm not constipated. I eliminate every day and I don't need a colon cleansing"?

Despite daily eliminations, many people are not aware that they may have a bowel problem. Very often, the complete length of the colon is impacted with old, hardened fecal matter, leaving only a narrow channel for smaller, softer feces to pass through. Failure to cleanse the colon is like having an entire garbage-collecting staff go on strike for months on end!

The colon is the sewage system of the body. If the wastes in the colon are allowed to build up, they will decay and absorb through the walls of the colon into the bloodstream. These toxins can poison the brain and nervous system so that you become depressed, irritable, weak, and listless; poison the lungs so that your breath is foul; poison the digestive system so that you are distressed and bloated; poison the blood so that your skin is sallow and unhealthy. In short, every organ is affected and you look and feel old, have stiff and painful joints, dull eyes, and sluggish thinking. Finally, you lose the joy of living. As Dr. Wager wrote about the Law of Disease:

Disease is a warning. It is a friend, not a foe, of mankind. It manifests itself in its various forms, from a slight cold to the more severe inflammations for the sole purpose of ridding the body of accumulated poisons.

Toxic Buildup

When people finally visit their doctor, they often have suffered for years from many of the following symptoms of toxic buildup and constipation:

- Fatigue and depression
- Gas-belching or flatulence
- Headaches
- Irritability, anxiety, nervousness
- Insomnia
- Nausea and abdominal discomfort

- Protruding, tender, or rigid abdomen
- Sagging posture
- Lack of interest in work or play
- Loss of memory or concentration
- Lack of sexual response
- Overweight, underweight, poor appetite, malnutrition
- Skin blemishes, sallow complexion, dark circles under the eyes
- Brittle hair and nails
- Bad breath, coated tongue, body odors
- Cold hands and feet
- Swelling of the legs
- Lower back pain
- Menstrual problems
- Blood pressure too high or too low
- Neuritis and neuralgia (aches and pains in different areas of the body)

Imbalances of the Colon

Structural, functional, and metabolic imbalances of the colon are manifested in various forms. The effects of autointoxication and constipation are shown in the most common abnormalities of the colon, such as adhesions, ballooning, colitis, diverticulitis, mucosal dysfunction, spastic or irritated bowel, strictures, and ulceration.

The following drawings illustrate the various abnormal shapes of the bowel in comparison to a normal bowel.

No doubt should exist about the relation between health of the intestinal tract and health in the rest of the body. Intestinal management probably is the most important factor a person can learn in a health-building routine. Some of the most important functions of life take place in the intestines. There, worn-out cells are eliminated and new cell structures are begun.

Normal and Abnormal Colons

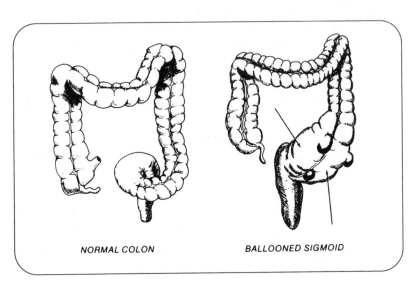

NORMAL COLON   BALLOONED SIGMOID

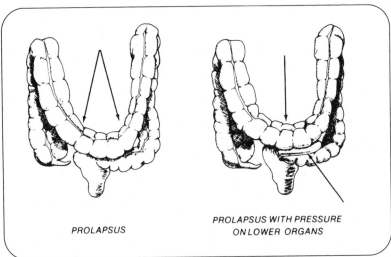

PROLAPSUS

PROLAPSUS WITH PRESSURE
ON LOWER ORGANS

Reprinted by permission of Bernard Jensen, D.C., Ph.D., from his book *Tissue Cleansing through Bowel Management*, 1981.

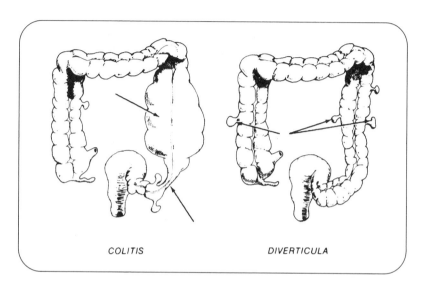

COLITIS   DIVERTICULA

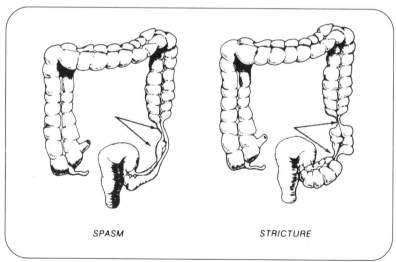

SPASM   STRICTURE

Attitudes that Promote Intestinal Inefficiency

By putting the bowel in the closet and making believe it doesn't exist, many people have gone down the path of improper living, treating the bowel indiscriminately and reaping the sad harvest in later years.

—Bernard Jensen, D.C., Ph.D.

Although incredible quantities of laxatives and stimulants are consumed by the general public each year, with or without professional advice or supervision (mostly without), the causes of intestinal problems are rarely examined. This unfortunate condition arises from the following viewpoints:

- A credulous public acceptance of many medical authorities who maintain that "Your bowels—like the universe—will get along very well if you leave them alone. They will adjust themselves to the body they inhabit and the kind of food you eat."
- A belief that constipation is an unimportant symptom, easily relieved by taking laxatives, bran, stimulants or other ineffective solutions to the real problem.

Causes of Constipation

- Too little liquid
- Too little bulk
- Too little exercise
✓ • Parasites
✓ • Yeast overgrowth (candida)
✓ • Emotional tension
- Mechanical problems, e.g., a prolapsed colon
- Poor choice of foods
- Improper combination of foods
- Temperature of foods too hot or too cold
- Weak muscle tone of the colon
- Inherited weaknesses

Constipating Foods and Drinks

- Cheese
- Fried foods
- Candies and sugar products
- White flour
- Salt
- Salted snack foods (potato chips, etc.)
- Beef
- Canned, burned, fermented or processed foods
- Heavy, hardshelled or cellulose foods, such as tops of vegetables and legumes
- Pasteurized milk
- Wine with meals
- Carbonated drinks
- Coffee (has a drying effect on the colon)

If you are consuming these foods and drinks, your colon cannot possibly be healthy, even if you are having a bowel movement every day. Instead of furnishing nourishment to the nerves, muscle cells, and tissues of the walls of the colon, such substances can actually cause starvation of the colon. A starved colon may let a lot of fecal matter pass through it, but it is unable to carry on the last stages of digestion. Remember, cancer of the colon ranks next to heart disease as the most frequent cause of death in our country.

In order to be healthy, the body must be nourished properly. The colon produces a coat of mucous to protect itself from junk foods, pasteurized milk, preservatives, chemicals, and other pollutants. In time, this mucous coating can get as thick and hard as plastic. You can spend a fortune on vitamins, herbs, and organic foods, but the mucous coating prevents proper absorption of nutrients into your bloodstream. Colon cleansing does much to remove the excess mucous and eliminate a toxic buildup from lining the walls of the colon. After a series of colon cleansings, you will experience a greater joy of living as well as a greater understanding of how this important system functions.

Attitudes that Promote Health

It is with love and self-respect that you establish for yourself a balanced lifestyle that promotes greater health. This includes cleansing the colon on a regular basis, exercise, fresh air, stress-release activities (meditation, massage, having fun), getting ample rest, drinking plenty of water, and eliminating drugs, processed foods, foods grown with pesticides, sugar, coffee, and other agents of disease from your diet.

Many people turn to colon cleansing when they find themselves in a state of disease or pain. Why not do so out of a desire to cleanse the body in order to achieve greater strength, mental awareness, and a sense of well-being? Knowing that you are in control of your body is the most important step toward realizing your health goals.

In his article "Gastrointestinal Therapy in Atrophic Arthritis," E. Goldfain, M.D., outlines his concepts for maintaining the digestive tract at its best.

A proper food supply: Adequate vitamins and minerals must be present, especially calcium, phosphorus, and iron.

Good intestinal drainage: This is of paramount importance. If the bowel, especially the colon, is to function adequately, the amount and type of food that is ingested must be such as to avoid an excessive burden on the intestinal tract. If the bulk of ingested food does not overload the lower digestive system, then the colon will automatically function more effectively. As Dr. Bernard Jensen tells us:

Bowel cleansing is an essential element in any lasting healing program. The toxic waste must be removed as quickly as possible to halt this downward spiral of failing health.

Colon Reflex Chart

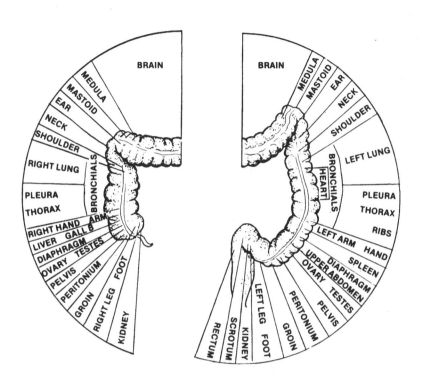

The colon produces reflex conditions in various organs in the body. In the above chart, the organ opposite the particular part of the bowel shows the part of the body affected directly by the colon. Symptoms in various parts of the body are relieved and many times eliminated when the intestinal flora have been changed. No matter what conditions we have in the body, they are affected by the bowel whether it is good or bad.

Reprinted from *Science and Practice of Iridology*, by Bernard Jensen, D.C., N.D., Escondido, CA, 1952.

2

Suggestions to Improve Bowel Function

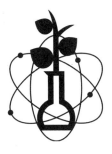

Suggestions to Improve Bowel Function

In addition to colon cleansing, you can improve your bowel function and feeling of well-being by consuming the proper foods and liquids, combining and cooking foods correctly, and exercising and meditating regularly.

- At least 50 percent of the foods you eat should be "live"—fresh, raw, and unprocessed (preferably organic). Dead foods cannot build strong bodies. Eat foods in season.
- Have your main meal as early in the day as possible. Eat two-thirds of your daily intake before mid-afternoon. Do not go to sleep at night on a full stomach.
- Chew your food well; at least 10 to 20 chews for each mouthful.
- Do not eat if ill or emotionally upset; do not overeat.
- Eat the following daily: six vegetables, two fruits, one starch, and one protein. Vary these foods from meal to meal and from day to day.
- Eat at least one full serving of a whole grain daily, such as millet, brown rice, or yellow cornmeal.
- Eat at least two full servings of raw or cooked vegetables daily, including one serving of such vegetables as cabbage, brussels sprouts, or sauerkraut.

- Eat foods (greens) containing potassium and sodium.
- Eat two ounces of fresh sprouts daily: bean, mung, fenugreek, pea.
- Eat at least one pound of raw fruit daily: apples, bananas, papaya, pineapple, figs, dates, prunes. Always soak dried fruit overnight in apple juice and eat for breakfast.
- Eat at least one pint of yogurt daily, preferably goat yogurt. Also add kefir (not sweetened with sugar) to your diet.
- Eat one ounce of unfiltered honey daily with yogurt or tea.
- Eat lots of fibrous foods.

Liquids To Improve Bowel Function

- Drink sufficient liquids (water, juices, herbal teas): one-half ounce daily for each pound of body weight. For example, if you weigh 128 pounds, you should drink 64 ounces (8 cups) of liquids daily.
- Do not drink liquids with meals. Take liquids between meals using distilled or filtered water, unsweetened juices, herbal teas, or grain beverages.
- Drink eight ounces of goat milk daily. Warm the milk and sip it slowly.

Food Combining and Amounts

- Select 70 percent of your daily food intake from alkaline-forming foods; 30 percent from acid-forming foods.
- It's easier on your digestive system if you do not eat fruits and vegetables at the same meal. Have fruit for breakfast and a mid-afternoon snack.
- Starch and protein do not combine well. Have one at lunch, the other at dinner. It's best to eat protein in the morning and at noon, rather than in the evening.

Alkaline-Forming Foods
Fruit juices, goat's milk, vegetable juices, potatoes, fruits, vegetables, raw honey, sprouting seeds.

Acid-Forming Foods
Meat, fish, fowl, cheese, eggs, rice, bread, cereal, peanuts, nuts, sugar (avoid), citrus juices.

Foods To Avoid or Replace

- Avoid nuts or peanut butter.
- Avoid very hot or very cold food or liquids.
- Eliminate fried foods of all kinds; instead, bake, broil, or steam your foods.
- Avoid pork and pork products (lunch meats, hot dogs, ham, bacon, etc.). Many parasites in pork are heat resistant.
- If you are a red-meat eater, reduce your daily intake to two ounces or less. Replace red meat with fish or fowl whenever possible. Always purchase poultry, beef, and other animal products that haven't been fed antibiotics and growth hormones. These additives destroy the vital intestinal flora, are carcinogenic, and damage bowel function. Many health food stores now carry range-fed poultry. The cost is slightly higher but well worth the price difference.
- Replace table salt (NaCl) with Dr. Jensen's Seasoning Powder or Bio-Salt. If you must use salt, use sea salt (naturally evaporated) rather than iodized salt.

Cooking Suggestions

- Do not use aluminum or Teflon™ cookware because tiny particles of metal or coatings chip off and leach into the food. Also, the oxidation process of cooking in aluminum is harmful to foods. Use stainless steel whenever possible.

- Do not wrap food in aluminum foil unless the food is first wrapped in plastic.
- Cook with low heat; cook with little water and cover the pan. Cook vegetables as little as possible. Crock pots will retain a majority of nutrients in food.
- Do not fry foods; instead, bake, broil or steam them.

Bowel Function

- Take all laxatives out of your medicine cabinet and throw them away.
- The most beneficial time of day for bowel elimination is early in the morning, either before or soon after breakfast.
- Make a habit to try to have a bowel movement first thing in the morning, whether you receive the call or not. Allow at least 15 minutes; do not strain. Remember, weak bowels take more time to function. Breathing deeply and bending the head toward the knees while in the sitting or squatting position can help.
- Take pleasure and pride in your bowel health.

Exercise and Meditation

- Develop some form of deep-breathing and meditation exercises.
- Express your feelings more—loosen up! Constipation can be associated with the refusal to release old ideas. Try this affirmation each day: "I release the past. I generously allow life to flow through me."
- Do plenty of exercise daily: walking, running, jumping, bending, stretching, yoga, self-massage, and slant-board exercises.

Slant-Board Exercises

For Prolapsed Colon and Regenerating
the Vital Nerve Centers of the Brain

by Bernard Jensen, D.C., Ph.D.

Slant-board exercises are absolutely necessary to regaining perfect health. These exercises are a vital means to increase blood flow to the brain, tone the muscles, and improve circulation to all areas of the body.

When there is a lack of tone in the muscles of the colon, you can expect prolapsus (a dropping) of the abdominal organs. If the body lacks tone, the heart cannot circulate blood properly. Likewise, arteries and veins cannot contract to help move the blood against gravity into the brain tissues.

Slant-board exercises are practically the same as any other lying-down exercises and are especially good in cases of inflammations and congestions above the neck. This includes sinus trouble, failing eyesight, hair loss, head eczema, ear conditions, and similar problems. Slant-board exercises have helped in cases of heart trouble, fatigue, dizziness, poor memory, and paralysis.

There are some people who have tried nearly everything to get well and who still find all organs working under par. Many people do not realize that all the quickening force for every organ of the body comes from the brain. The heart gets its start from the brain and continues its everlasting pumping because of it. People whose occupations require them to sit or stand continually are unable to get the blood into the brain tissues because the tired organs cannot force the blood uphill. If the brain tissues are denied good blood in the proper amount, in time every organ in the body will suffer.

There are some cases where the slant board is contra-indicated. It is usually best to get professional advice, for some people have had unhappy experiences because they started with too strenuous a program. If you haven't done much exercising of the abdominal muscles, it is well to take these exercises slowly and gradually increase them as you get stronger.

Do not use the board in cases of high blood pressure, hemorrhages, some tubercular conditions, cancer in the pelvic cavity, appendicitis, ulcers of the stomach or intestines, or pregnancy, unless under the care of a physician.

Directions for Using the Slant Board

Rest the head end of the board on the floor and put the foot end at chair height for all exercises. If you become dizzy at first, don't raise the foot end of the board quite so high to begin with.

In the beginning, do slant-board exercises only five minutes a day; more than that is too much. As you become more accustomed to the exercises, gradually increase time spent on the board.

The following numbered exercises correspond to the following illustrations.

1. Lie full length, allowing gravity to help the abdominal organs into their position. For best results, lie on the board at least 10 minutes, preferably at mid-afternoon and again just before going to bed. After retiring, lift the buttocks up to allow the organs to return to their normal position.
2. While lying flat on your back, stretch the abdomen by putting arms above head. Bring arms above head 10 to 15 times; this stretches the abdominal muscles and pulls the abdomen down toward the shoulders.

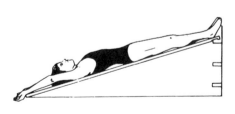

1

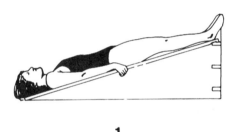

2

3. Bring abdominal organs toward shoulders while holding your breath. Move the organs back and forth by drawing them upward, contracting abdominal muscles, and then allowing them to go back to a relaxed position. Do this 10 to 15 times.
4. Pat abdomen vigorously with open hands. Lean to one side, then to the other, patting the stretched side. Pat 10 to 15 times each side.

Bring the body to sitting position, using the abdominal muscles. Return to lying position. Do this three to four times, if possible. Do only if your doctor orders.

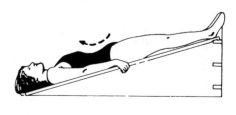

3

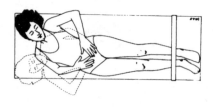

4

Hold on to the sides of the board while doing the following exercises.

5. Bend knees and legs at hips. While in this position
   (a) turn head from side to side five or six times, and
   (b) lift head slightly and rotate in circles three or four times.
6. Lift legs to vertical position, rotate outward in circles eight or ten times. Increase to 25 times after a week or two of exercising.

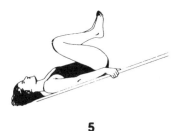

5

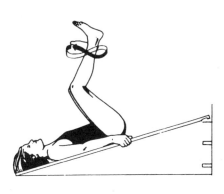

6

7. Bring legs straight up to a vertical position and lower them to the board slowly. Repeat three or four times.
8. Bicycle legs in air 15 to 25 times.
   Relax and rest, letting blood circulate in the head for 10 minutes.

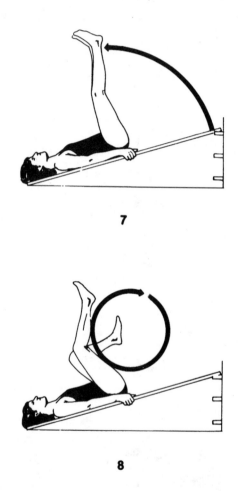

7

8

Reprinted by permission of Bernard Jensen, D.C., Ph.D., from his book *Tissue Cleansing through Bowel Management,* 1981.

The Ileocecal Valve Syndrome

by Dr. David G. Williams

Every so often I run into a technique or method of helping people that is so dramatic and simple to use that I wish the whole world could be aware of it. Techniques involving the ileocecal valve (ill-lee-o-see-cal) are a good example of this.

Wouldn't it be nice to know something to do when you or your family had a sudden case of diarrhea or constipation? Or wouldn't it be nice to stop those so-called flu-type symptoms that so often hit with absolutely no warning? When the ileocecal valve isn't working right, it can cause these symptoms and many more. Just look at the list of things that it can cause:

- shoulder pain
- nausea
- dizziness
- chest pains
- heart fluttering
- bursitis-like pain in the shoulders and hip joints
- light-headedness
- ringing in the ear
- lower back pain for no reason
- recurrent sinus infections
- headaches and fever

What and Where Is This Valve?

The ileocecal valve is located between the small and large intestine. Basically, it is located in the same area as the appendix and many times what is thought to be an appendix problem is instead a problem with the valve. This little valve has two very important jobs to do. First, it serves as a block that prevents the toxic contents of the large intestine from backing up into the small intestine. Second, it keeps the food products in the small intestine from passing into the large intestine before the digestive processes have been completed.

The valve can at times become either stuck shut or stuck open. When stuck shut, the ileocecal valve can cause constipation, and when stuck open, diarrhea will be the problem.

31

When the Valve Sticks Shut

Food becomes toxic after staying in the body too long. It should move on through the large intestine and then be expelled by the body. Sometimes, if the valve sticks shut, the feces or toxic waste material will have to stay in the small intestine and will be unable to move any further. Naturally, since the small intestine's job is to absorb, it keeps right on working and absorbing all of the waste products and garbage into the body! Also, with the valve shut and the food backing up, you become constipated.

When the Valve Sticks Open

By sticking open, the ileocecal valve not only allows food to move through you at a rapid rate (to say the least), but it also lets the waste products in the large intestine back up into the small intestine and again be reabsorbed into the system!

It doesn't take a genius to realize that the valve can cause a world of problems, but better yet, it doesn't take a genius to do some easy things to help stabilize the valve.

Why Me?

There are several reasons why the valve doesn't always work right, but I'll only mention a few of the more common ones here. Sometimes spicy or roughage-type foods will irritate the valve and cause it to stick shut or open. Another factor that greatly influences the valve is stress or emotional trauma. Almost everyone is exposed to these factors, but some of us are more sensitive than others. I personally find that those who have had their appendix removed seem to have more problems. Some researchers believe that the appendix, which is located right next to the valve, acts like "an overflow bag for toxins" and holds these until the body can work them slowly and not interrupt the workings of the ileocecal valve.

Open Ileocecal Valve—What to Do

When the valve is open (diarrhea, loose stools, and symptoms like those mentioned earlier), there are some temporary things that can be done first. The valve is located on the right side, about halfway between the belly button and the hip bone. Many times you can get relief in one of two ways.

First, you can sometimes hold the valve shut for several minutes. This is done by placing your hand over the valve and while pushing in, pull up toward the left shoulder.

The second way is to place a cold pack made of cold water or ice over the valve for about 15 to 20 minutes. This process can be repeated if necessary.

Stopping the Flu Dead in Its Tracks

Except for the two things to do for diarrhea and an open ileocecal valve (which I also find works quite well for travelers in Mexico who are suffering from the famous so-called tourista or Montezuma's revenge), there are several things that need to be done for both the open and the closed valve.

When I find this problem with one of my patients or if I have a patient suffering from either diarrhea or constipation, I instruct the patient as follows:

1. First, the toxic food products that are either backing up or that are blocked up in the intestines need to be detoxified and the best method to do this is to use either garlic or chlorophyll. I find that chlorophyll works best and is easy to obtain at any health food store. Initially, either two capsules or tablets or one half teaspoon of chlorophyll liquid should be taken every two hours for about six to eight hours and the same amount with each meal for the next three to four days.

2. Next, the diet should be modified to eliminate spicy foods for a week or so. If the problem is diarrhea, it is also helpful to eliminate all roughage-type food for a short

CHAPTER 2

period of time. If the ileocecal valve is closed and constipation is a problem, then increase the roughage.

3. Alcohol, cocoa, chocolate, and caffeine products should be eliminated.
4. With a closed valve (constipation), add calcium and vitamin D to the diet.
5. With an open valve (diarrhea), add to the diet a product called lactic acid yeast, which can be obtained at any health food store. This product alone can sometimes stop even the most stubborn cases of chronic diarrhea.
6. MOST IMPORTANT OF ALL, BY RUBBING ON THE FOLLOWING "REFLEX" POINTS FOR BOTH THE OPEN AND THE CLOSED ILEOCECAL VALVE, YOU CAN RELIEVE THE PROBLEM ALMOST INSTANTLY!

The areas illustrated in the diagram on page 35 should be massaged with firm pressure for about 10 to 20 seconds each (it is not beneficial to rub the points any longer than that; in fact, it may negate the effect).

Most of the points will be extremely sore if the problem is long standing. Ask a cooperative friend to work out the points, or use a vibrator.

The next time you first start to get the flu-like symptoms of achiness, fatigue or sore throat, or the next time you or a member of your family start to have problems with either constipation or diarrhea, try rubbing on these reflex points. You might be surprised to find that your problem may leave in a matter of minutes instead of weeks!

Reprinted from *Alternatives,* Vol. 1, No. 3, a monthly health newsletter written by Dr. David G. Williams, published by Mountain Home Publishing, P.O. Box 829, Ingram, TX 78025. Subscription price $39 per year.

Ileocecal Valve Reflex Points

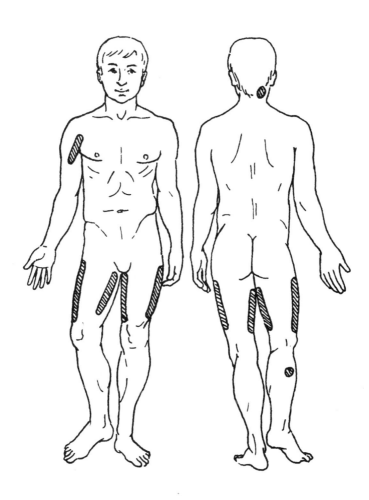

The areas illustrated should be massaged with firm pressure for about *10 to 20 seconds* each (it is not beneficial to rub the points any longer than that; in fact, it may negate the effect).

3

Colon Therapy: Pathway to Vibrant Health

Although colon health emphasizes prevention, many people have found relief from constipation, fatigue, poor eyesight, hearing loss, asthma, prostate trouble, colds, allergies, nagging backache, respiratory disorders, digestive problems, gas, abdominal pain, colitis, indigestion, overweight, nutritional deficiencies, hypoglycemia, depression, anxiety, tenseness, and numerous other ailments.

—Norman W. Walker, D.Sc.

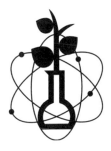

Benefits of Colon Therapy

Colon therapy is a restorative, relaxing experience that is both pleasant and effective. Most people report relief of problems after the very first treatment. Vitality and energy levels are restored. Colon therapy has an antiseptic and solvent action on the intestines, whereby putrefactive material, impacted fecal matter, excess mucous, and even pus and infected tissue are removed from the colon. This leaves a cleaner, healthier colon, which means a healthier body.

Colon therapy increases the water level and diuretic action of the body. Water is absorbed into the body, which increases the volume of the blood. Circulation is thereby increased, resulting in greater bathing of the individual cells, thus diluting toxins and flushing them out; relieving uremia and toxemia; and increasing elimination both through kidneys and skin as well as the bowel. All this generally assists the cardiovascular and circulatory systems' efficiency.

During a colon cleansing, both warm and cool water may be used. The warm water supplies heat to the body. The cleansing action along with the warm temperature is excellent for relieving colds and flu. Probably the greatest benefit of bathing the colon in warm water is relief from tension and irritability. X-rays following treatment demonstrate that spastic colons are more relaxed and relieved of muscle spasms as well as the swelling, irritation, and inflammation of tissues that accompany this problem.

On the other hand, the effects of cool water can also be beneficial. Any time there is a fever, cool water will aid in reducing it. Swollen tissues can be alleviated and a loose or elongated colon can also be improved. A colon lacking tone, accompanied by gas and constipation, will benefit greatly by the stimulation of the cleansing. This stimulation induces peristalsis, the wavelike muscular contractions and dilations of the colon that move the contents forward.

Many colon X-rays show that pressure of constipation is exerted in the liver area, resulting in irritation to both liver and gall bladder, as well as to the common bile duct. This delays and obstructs the normal draining of these organs—a condition that is often alleviated through colon therapy.

In some cases, pain in the heart area is also relieved. X-rays demonstrate that parts of the colon can be very high in the upper left quadrant causing irritation to the heart. Rapid heartbeat, hypertension, and various chest pains may all be alleviated by proper intestinal cleansing.

Many overweight patients have eliminated as much as 10 to 25 pounds by having their intestinal tract cleansed. Constipation is responsible for the accumulation of large amounts of fecal matter in that area as well as allowing the body wastes to build up at the cellular level. Proper colon cleansing aids greatly in eliminating unwanted and unsightly excess pounds—not to mention that dull, irritable feeling that is so prevalent. Unfortunately, weight gain comes upon people so gradually that they often don't realize what changes occur from year to year.

Various other results are often seen. Some patients report they have never been able to perspire until receiving colon therapy. Because of the removal of toxic wastes, the skin becomes strong and healthy and people look years younger. Memory is often improved. A feeling of well-being hastens the removal of

Six Colon X-Rays

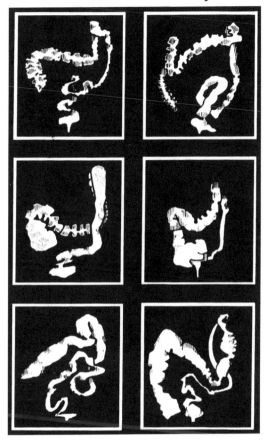

The above six pictures of prolapsed, distorted, twisted, sickly-looking colons are exact reproductions of X-ray negatives of the colons of apparently healthy, civilized people whose illusions about their physical condition were exploded when they saw this conclusive evidence.

Civilized life means an artificial life; civilized people, living in a civilized manner and eating civilized foods, cannot, in the very nature of things, have a truly healthy colon.

Health and sickness both have their roots in the colon.

—Dr. Norman W. Walker, D.Sc.

bowel contents (mucous, gas, parasites, undigested food particles, glandular and cellular debris, plus bacterial toxins).

Gentle abdominal massage during a colon cleansing helps release fecal impactions, moving the water around to help break up the solidified crust on the inner surface of the colon. It also stimulates peristalsis and helps return the colon to its normal shape, thus removing pressure on other organs (liver, gall bladder, stomach, heart, etc.). Dr. Bernard Jensen wrote:

> Every person who desires the higher things in life must be aware of proper bowel management, what it is, how it works, and what is required. In so doing, you will discover many secrets of life, develop a positive attitude toward yourself, and become the master of body function.

Colon Therapy with Oxygen

In recent years, a new approach to colon therapy has been introduced. By mixing medically pure oxygen with the water used to flush the colon, therapists have achieved miraculous results. Those patients who previously had colon cleansings report many differences in the results.

Colon therapy with oxygen has a definite calming effect on the nervous system. Nervousness and irritability are both lessened. A person not only becomes easier to live with, but feels so much better from both improved nerve functions and having eliminated toxins that irritate the nerves.

There is no comparison in the way one feels after a cleansing with the new procedure with oxygen. In fact, it is reported that the small blood vessels lining the colon instantly absorb oxygen—normalizing not only the lower bowel, but also the entire body. Some authorities state that, liter per liter, more oxygen is absorbed through colon cleansing than through the lungs. This not only helps to heal the affected tissues in the colon, but also allows the oxygen to pass quickly into the bloodstream and bathe all the cells in the body.

Oxygen aids in the healing of sores and wounds. In many

cases, acidophilus or lactobacilli (the friendly bacteria) have been destroyed by improper eating habits, constipation, diarrhea, parasites, an infected colon, and antibiotics. Affected areas in the colon, resulting in irritation, infection, colitis, ulceration, and diverticulosis are bathed with a continuous supply of their life-supporting element, oxygen, which hastens healing in the colon as well as other parts of the body.

Colon therapy with oxygen has an anthelmintic action; that is, parasites are removed. Many patients are found to have some form of parasites, the most common being tapeworm. Various other types found are hookworms, pinworms, roundworms, whipworms, and many other exotic forms. Sources of tapeworms are usually beef, pork or fish. Many vegetarians also are infected with various parasites by eating vegetables or fruit infested with parasite eggs. Dr. Norman Walker said:

> Experience has taught me that no health and healing procedures can be as successful as those which have a series of colon irrigations as the prelude to any health treatment. This makes sense because just so long as there is material in the colon which may be conducive to the generation of poisons in the colon and to the diffusion of such poisons throughout the system, no healing can take place which is not the precursor of a chain reaction of ailments at a future date.

Colon-Cleansing Procedure

A colon cleansing is a gentle, warm-water washing of the colon (large intestine) combined with some external massage. Also known as intestinal hydrotherapy or colonic irrigation, it is completely safe, beneficial, and nontoxic.

The procedure lasts approximately 45 minutes and is performed by a colon therapist using a colon irrigation machine that regulates the water pressure, temperature, and water volume. A five-inch speculum attached to a hose (both disposable) is inserted into the anus, allowing the water to flow in under gentle pressure to cleanse the entire length of the colon. The water dislodges toxic wastes in the colon, which are then flushed out through the waste hose. During a cleansing, a series of water-fills and releases also helps to stimulate the expansion and contraction of the muscular walls of the colon. This, combined with a changing of the water temperature from warm to cool, exercises the colon and promotes the restoration of proper peristaltic action.

During the cleansing, most people find that they can relax completely. After the cleansing is completed, acidophilus can be taken orally to increase the level of beneficial flora present in the intestinal tract.

Note: Since nearly all tap water contains chemicals as well as other undesirable substances, it is most important that the water used in a colon cleansing be purified by some form of filtration system.

Most up-to-date colonic machines are equipped with disposable hoses and speculums to insure cleanliness. You should insist on disposable accessories that are used only once and then thrown away.

Commonly Asked Questions about Colon Therapy

Q: Are colon cleansings completely safe?

A: Yes. In fact, with the latest colonic equipment (an oxygen-equipped colon cleansing machine), treatments are much safer than the common enema.

Q: How does a colon cleansing compare to an enema?

A: An enema only bathes the lower part of the colon, whereas a colon cleansing bathes the entire length of the colon, approximately five to five and a half feet. A colon cleansing is many more times effective, according to learned centenarian Dr. Norman Walker, who said, "One colonic is equivalent to 30 enemas."

Q: Can I be constipated even if I have 1, 2 or 3 bowel movements a day?

A: Yes. Accumulated wastes, mucous and gas in the colon may inhibit its natural peristaltic action, resulting in incomplete—though frequent—bowel movements.

Q: How many times do I need to take a colonic?

A: Often the waste is so hard and deeply lodged in the colon that it may take a series of colonics to sufficiently soften and loosen it. Colonics also stimulate the liver, kidney and lymph system to dump toxins. The number of treatments varies with each individual and his/her condition. Your therapist can best advise you regarding this.

Q: Do treatments hurt?

A: No. In fact, with the advanced equipment now available, treatments are refreshing and relaxing.

Q: Are colonics habit-forming?

A: No. The purpose of cleansing the colon is to allow it to relax and rejuvenate and promote better peristalsis. The colon cannot heal when it is constantly working to get rid of accumulated wastes, gases and poisons.

Q: How much of the intestines are actually cleansed during a colon cleansing?

A: During a treatment we are actually able to bathe the full length of the colon, but we are not able to cleanse the small intestine. The buildup in the small intestine is cleared with the help of the Intestinal Cleanser and other nutritional aids taken orally during a series of cleansings.

Q: Should I see my doctor before having a colon cleansing?

A: If there is something organically or internally wrong, it's always a good idea to consult your doctor. However, since colon cleansings professionally administered with the new colon hydrotherapy equipment are safer than home enemas, a medical examination is not required except for those who are ill.

Q: How long does a treatment take?

A: Between 40 to 50 minutes, but you should plan for an hour stay.

Q: Does having a menstrual period at the time of the cleanse have any effect on the success of the treatment?

A: No, in fact it's usually a good time to receive a treatment, since your body is already cleansing. Your menstrual flow will not interfere with the success of the treatment. Flushing the colon will also reduce abdominal pressure associated with menstrual cycles.

Q: What should I do to prepare for a colon cleansing?

A: Refrain from eating before the cleansing, be as relaxed as possible, and maintain a positive, cheerful attitude. Do not drink carbonated beverages, because they will add gas to the colon.

Q: Is there any possibility of bacterial or viral contamination from prior use of the colonic machine?

A: That's a very timely question. The latest colonic machines now use presterilized disposable hoses and speculums. Since these accessories are *only used once* and then thrown away, there is no danger of contamination.

Q: Will I experience any intestinal discomfort or fatigue after the cleansing?

A: Not usually, but since the cleansing will stir up a lot of old debris and toxins, you might experience some nausea or fatigue. I recommend resting and applying a warm heating pad to the abdomen if any discomfort occurs. A mild vegetable broth or peppermint tea is usually soothing at this time. Any discomfort will usually pass within 24 hours.

Q: Won't colonics damage the normal intestinal flora?

A: Accumulation of encrusted feces in the colon makes it impossible for the glands to produce the necessary intestinal flora, resulting in increased constipation. Cleansing the colon helps bring the acid-alkaline ratio back into balance, allowing friendly bacteria to thrive, while inhibiting disease-causing organisms. You can assist the body in this process by orally taking acidophilus to reintroduce friendly bacteria into the colon. I recommend taking acidophilus capsules during a cleansing program and continuing for at least 60 days afterward. (See Chapter 5 for more information on acidophilus.)

Q: Can I work after a colon cleansing?
A: Certainly. Colon cleansing should not interfere with your scheduled day.

Q: I always had a well functioning colon and I would have at least one bowel movement a day. Lately, I am not having success every day and I am experiencing some gas and bloating. When I do have a bowel movement, it is usually soft or in pieces. Sometimes, it will get very hard or very soft. What is my problem?
A: Changeable stools plus periods of gas and bloating may be a signal of parasites or candida overgrowth. Be sure to read Chapters 6 and 7 on these subjects.

Note: If you are interested in pursuing a career in colon therapy, or are seeking a colon therapist in your area, call Ray Dotolo at (800) 237-5911 for more information. The companies manufacturing professional equipment are:
• Dotolo Research: (800) 237-5911
• Specialty Health Products: (602) 582-4950

4

Healing Within Four- or Seven-Day Colon Cleansing Program

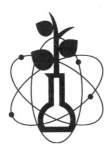

Healing Within *Four-* or *Seven-Day* *Colon Cleansing Program*

Colon cleansing treatments are the central focus of this program, since so much toxic buildup accumulates in the organs of elimination. The colon cleansing treatments remove much of the old waste material and mucous buildup. These treatments will help cleanse your elimination organs: the skin, kidneys, lungs, liver, bowel, and lymphatic system. The cleansing program is not represented as a cure for any disease or ailment. It is simply a method of cleansing the body to help create a healthier YOU.

The cleanse is not to be considered a weight-loss program, but it is not unusual to lose five to seven pounds during the course of the four to seven days. Since the cleansing process helps improve digestion, assimilation, and elimination, additional weight loss may occur even when you return to solid foods.

Please observe as closely as possible all instructions and the suggested schedule on the following pages. Each product and procedure has its purpose and should produce wonderful results.

Note: I do not recommend that you attempt this program without some form of colon cleansing. Enemas are helpful, but colonics work best and are more thorough. Visit your colon therapist as recommended. If you need to locate a therapist in your area, call Ray Dotolo at (800) 237-5911 for information.

The program will seldom conflict with any other therapy or treatment, but if you are presently under a doctor's care, it is best to discuss this program with your physician and seek his or her counsel and support. If your doctor is interested in preventive health care, he or she will understand that a clean body will be more responsive to any therapeutic measures that you may need.

The program is not intended to replace qualified medical care. I recommend that the seriously ill and the elderly go easy with this program, seeking the advice of their doctor in modifying any of these procedures to conform to individual specific needs and limitations.

Instructions

The following is a step-by-step instruction guide for the Four- or Seven-Day Colon Cleansing Program.

If you are doing the Four-Day Cleansing Program, you should begin all products on Day 1. You should receive colon cleansings on Days 2, 3, and 4 of the program.

If you are doing the Seven-Day Cleansing Program, you should begin all products on Day 1. You should receive colon cleansings on Days 2, 3, 5, and 7 of the program.

- Eat nothing else during the cleansing program other than what is specified in these instructions.
- Discontinue all vitamin and mineral supplements during the cleansing program.
- Drink distilled, bottled, or filtered water (6 to 8 glasses daily), herbal teas, Bernard Jensen's broth, and diluted fresh vegetable and fruit juices. Lots of liquids are essential for best results. Avoid orange, pineapple, and grapefruit juices at this time, due to their high acid content. Do not drink canned, artificially flavored, or carbonated beverages during the cleansing program.

- Exercise moderately every day. The best exercise is a brisk walk, but always use good judgment and don't push yourself if you're fatigued.
- Avoid TV and movies at this time. Body cleansings are quiet times and are excellent opportunities to catch up on reading or listening to soothing music.
- Get a good night's rest, at least eight hours of sleep.
- Begin all products and procedures on the morning of Day 1. Your first colon cleansing will be on Day 2.

Products and Procedures

Apple Cider Vinegar Drink

Apple cider vinegar contains lots of potassium and is helpful in relieving mucous from the body. It is important to drink it immediately after you take the Colon 8 Intestinal Cleanser caplets.

Instructions: Mix 1 tablespoon of apple cider vinegar with 8 ounces of hot water. You may add a teaspoon of maple syrup if desired. Stir and drink at a moderate temperature. Follow it with an 8-ounce glass of water. (If you are afflicted with candida, you may want to avoid vinegar and syrup during this cleanse.)

Castor Oil Packs for the Immune System

Edgar Cayce, an acclaimed health practitioner, recommended castor oil packs in thousands of his psychic health readings. Although there has never been an extensive study of the medicinal effects of castor oil packs, it has been found that applying this oil as a heat pack on the abdomen has a profound relaxing and regenerative effect on the whole body. Beneficial results can be seen in the lymphatic system. Many of Cayce's recorded case histories indicate marvelous results. Cayce also recommended these packs be applied on nights before colon cleansings to relax and tone the colon.

Instructions: Gather together several large plastic garbage bags, several towels, a heating pad, a bowl, and the castor oil. Pour four ounces of castor oil into the bowl and soak the flannel cloth in the oil. Spread a plastic garbage bag on your bed with a towel on top of it and lie down on the towel.

Apply the cloth evenly to the general region of your abdomen. Next, put another large garbage bag over the cloth and tuck the bag under you. Place a towel over the plastic and apply the heating pad. Leave on for 1 to 1½ hours on low heat.

When this is completed, place the flannel cloth in a plastic bag and store it in the refrigerator. Apply the castor oil pack each evening before the day of the colon cleansing.

If you are on the Four-Day Cleansing Program, apply the castor oil pack on the evenings of Days 1, 2, and 3.

If you are on the Seven-Day Cleansing Program, apply the castor oil pack on the evenings of Days 1, 2, 4, and 6.

Colon 8 Intestinal Cleanser

This is a very important part of the cleansing program. Colon 8 Intestinal Cleanser is a mixture of herbs that scrubs and cleanses both the small intestine and the colon (large intestine). It will remove buildup of undigested food and mucous that may be lining the digestive and elimination system.

Instructions: Take 6 Colon 8 Intestinal Cleanser caplets 3 times a day.

DDS Acidophilus Culture

DDS Acidophilus culture is one of just a few brands of acidophilus that is acid resistant and can survive the long journey through the digestive tract to the colon. DDS delivers one billion friendly bacteria in each capsule. These bacteria will colonize and reestablish the much needed friendly flora that may be absent due to past antibiotic use. DDS helps improve bowel movements and also has an excellent cleansing effect on the liver. Acidophilus is also known to reduce blood cholesterol levels.

DDS should be taken with water only, the first thing in the morning and at bedtime. DDS should not be taken with food or other liquids because these substances would stimulate the natural stomach acids, which would weaken the ability of DDS to recolonize in the colon.

Instructions: Take 2 DDS Acidophilus capsules first thing in the morning and again at bedtime, with water only. Be sure to refrigerate the DDS Acidophilus capsules to keep the bacteria stable.

Dr. Jensen's Broth

This broth is loaded with vitamins and minerals. You will find it very satisfying during the cleansing, especially at dinner time. However, you can drink it as often as you wish. After your cleansing, try it as a substitute seasoning for salt and pepper. It is delicious on vegetables, salads, meat, or any cooked foods (do not use on fruit).

Instructions: Mix 1 teaspoon of Bernard Jensen's Broth with 8 ounces of hot water, stir, and drink.

Dry Skin Brushing

Dry skin brushing is the finest method I know to cleanse the skin. The skin should eliminate up to 2 pounds of wastes daily; skin brushing helps remove uric acid crystals, mucous, and other acids from the body. When the skin retains these waste materials, many of them are reabsorbed into the bloodstream. Brushing each day will keep your skin looking good and will reduce toxic buildup throughout your body.

You may find at first that the bristles feel very scratchy; this is normal. These are vegetable bristles and are not harmful to your skin. Just brush lightly until you become used to the sensation. After a few days, you will find that the brushing has stimulated your skin to take on a new glow. This should become a part of your daily hygiene, even after you complete this cleansing program.

Instructions: Brush the skin for 5 minutes in all directions over the body except the face. Brush first thing in the morning, before you shower or bathe.

Fresh Vegetable Juices

These are important during your cleansing program. Drink the vegetable juice as soon after juicing as possible, since raw juices will lose their enzyme value quickly. If you do not have a home juicer, stop at your health food store daily for raw juices. Some health food stores will make the juice fresh while you wait. Try to use organic vegetables for juicing whenever possible.

Instructions: Drink 4 ounces of vegetable juice mixed with 4 ounces of water, twice a day. I recommend a mixture of carrot, celery, beet, and parsley juices.

KB-11 Tablets

This is an excellent herbal combination to assist the kidneys in their function. It helps reduce water retention and aids in the elimination of uric acid and toxicity in very overworked kidneys.

Instructions: Take 2 tablets daily during the cleansing program.

OXY-OXC

OXY-OXC (pronounced "OX-ee-OX-ee") is an evolutionary breakthrough in oxygen nutrition. Through an advanced proprietary process, triatomic oxygen (Ozone) is bonded through a crystal lattice matrix with magnesium peroxide, allowing a multifaceted approach to cellular oxygenation. OXY-OXC is a body oxygenator and energizer which deetoxifies and cleanses wastes, pathogens and plaque from the gastro-intestinal tract, colon, arteries, and blood. For more information, see page 115 in Chapter 6.

Instructions: Take 2 capsules daily during the cleansing program.

Pau D'Arco Tea

This tea is made from tree bark imported from South America, where it has been in use for centuries. It has only recently received recognition in this country as a powerful healing tea and safe, natural antibiotic. It is very effective in reducing congestion throughout the lymph system as well as the lungs. It also helps clear mucous and acid buildup in the body. Pau D'Arco tea is a powerful aid for the immune system.

Instructions: Add 1 heaping tablespoon of Pau D'Arco tea bark to one quart of water. Bring to a boil and then simmer for 20 minutes. Strain off the bark, allow the tea to cool, and refrigerate. Drink no more than 8 ounces daily, hot or cold. You should continue to drink this tea after completing the cleansing program; make it a regular part of your diet.

Whole Life Food Blend

This nutritional whole food is a blend of chlorella, sesame seeds, colostrum, acidophilus, oat straw, and echinacea.

Chlorella's healing, cleansing and energizing power comes from its ability to rapidly concentrate sunlight and nutrients. It possesses 10 to 30 times more chlorophyll than alfalfa and is loaded with DNA, RNA and nucleic factors that speed up and intensify tissue repair, while increasing the supply of cellular nutrients.

Sesame seeds contain the oils and lecithin needed to feed the reproductive system, endocrine glands, nerves, and brain. High in protein, they also help prevent calcium loss from the bones.

Colostrum is high in immunoglobulins and nuclectides

which improve the immune system and colon functioning, while stimulating repair of tissues.

Oat straw has the power to regenerate and strengthen the nervous system while ridding the lungs of catarrh and keeping the joints flexible. Its silicon content improves the hair and nails and contributes to skin flexibility.

Echinacea is a cleanser, blood purifier and digestive aid which helps eliminate catarrh while benefiting the entire organic structure of the body.

Instructions: Add 1 teaspoon of Whole Life Food Blend to 4 ounces juice, preferably vegetable, and 4 ounces water. You may also use non-citrus fruit juices. Drink twice a day, once in the morning and once in the evening, and continue even after completing your fast. You can lose weight by skipping a meal and substituting Whole Life Food Blend in a glass of juice.

Four-Day Colon Cleansing Program

Day 1:   Begin all products. Follow *Suggested Time Schedule* on the following page.

Day 2:   Colon cleansing treatment. Continue with all products.

Day 3:   Colon cleansing treatment. Continue with all products.

Day 4:   Colon cleansing treatment. Use products up to the time of treatment. After the treatment discontinue Colon 8 Intestinal Cleanser, apple cider vinegar, KB-11 tablets, and castor oil packs.

Seven-Day Colon Cleansing Program

Day 1:   Begin all products. Follow the schedule below.

Day 2:   Colon cleansing treatment. Continue with all products.

Day 3:   Colon cleansing treatment. Continue with all products.

Day 4:   Continue with all products.

Day 5:   Colon cleansing treatment. Continue with all products.

Day 6:   Continue with all products.

Day 7:   Colon cleansing treatment. Use products up to the time of treatment. After the treatment discontinue Colon 8 Intestinal Cleanser, apple cider vinegar, KB-11 tablets, and castor oil packs.

Suggested Time Schedule

7:00 a.m.   **2 DDS Acidophilus** capsules with water only
5 Minutes Skin Brushing, then shower or bathe

7:15 a.m.   **6 Colon 8 Intestinal Cleanser caplets**
Apple Cider Vinegar Drink (1 tablespoon apple cider vinegar in 8 oz. hot water; add 1 teaspoon maple syrup if desired)
Glass of Water (8 oz.)

7:30 a.m.   **2 OXY-OXC capsules with 8 oz. water**

8:00 a.m.   **Pau D'Arco Tea** (8 oz.)

9:00 a.m.   **Whole Life Food Blend** in vegetable juice (1 teaspoon Food Blend, 4 oz. juice, 4 oz. water)

12:00 noon **Vegetable Juice** (4 oz. juice and 4 oz. water)

1:00 p.m.   **6 Colon 8 Intestinal Cleanser** caplets
Apple Cider Vinegar Drink
Glass of Water

3:00 p.m.   **2 KB-11 tablets**

5:00 p.m.   **Whole Life Food Blend** in vegetable juice and water

6:00 p.m.   **Dr. Jensen's Broth** (1 teaspoon broth in 8 oz. hot water)

8:00 p.m.   **6 Colon 8 Intestinal Cleanser Caplets**
Apple Cider Vinegar Drink
Glass of Water

8:30 p.m.   **Castor Oil Pack**

10:00 p.m. **2 DDS Acidophilus** capsules with water
Bedtime

Products Needed for the Colon Cleansing Program

You can order a kit containing the products you will need for this cleansing program by sending the order form beginning on page 291.

Products Supplied in Kit

Castor Oil (16 oz. liquid)
Colon 8 Intestinal Cleanser (120 caplets)
DDS Acidophilus (100 capsules)
Dr. Jensen's Broth (5 oz.)
Dry Skin Brush
Flannel Cloth (for castor oil application)
KB-11 (60 tablets)
OXY-OXC (180 capsules)
Pau D'Arco Tea (4 oz. bulk pkg.)
Whole Life Food Blend (16 oz.)

Products to Purchase at a Drugstore

Heating Pad

Products to Purchase at a Health Food Store

Apple Cider Vinegar (Hain's or Westbrae brands only)
Raw Apple Juice
Fresh Vegetable Juices
Pure Maple Syrup (optional)
Large Plastic Garbage Bags (grocery store)

Ending Your Colon Cleansing Program

Congratulations! You have completed your Four- or Seven-Day Colon Cleansing Program. Now that you have given your digestive and elimination systems a well-earned cleansing and rest, you are going to begin eating. Hopefully, you're feeling terrific. Here comes your first food test: ending your program properly by gradually introducing solid foods to your body. The key thought to remember is moderation! Applied to breaking a fast, this means consuming small quantities of food for the next few days.

Remember, any one can fast, but it takes wisdom to end a fast properly without sabotaging the good results achieved from this program. You can easily undo what you've done if you overeat at this time. Go slowly!

After your last colon cleansing, stop using the following products:

Apple Cider Vinegar Drink

Castor Oil Packs

Colon 8 Intestinal Cleanser

KB-11 Tablets

All the other products can be continued. I recommend that you continue drinking one cup of Pau D'Arco Tea daily. Take 2 DDS Acidophilus capsules with water first thing in the morning and just before bedtime for 30 days. Take 2 OXY-OXC capsules in the morning at least 5 minutes before eating. Continue Bernard Jensen's Broth as desired. Have a glass of fresh vegetable juice daily with a teaspoon of Whole Life Food Blend mixed in; there's no better way to get concentrated nutrition.

Try to avoid orange, pineapple, and grapefruit juices; they are hard on the kidneys and high in acids.

Dry brush your skin every day; 5 minutes brushing before bathing in the morning will make your skin glow with health.

Food Time

First Day

Breakfast: It's best to end your fast with a specially chosen fruit on the day after your last colon cleansing. Pre-select the fruit a day or so before, so it is ready and ripe for your first breakfast. Try to select an organic fruit if possible. The best choice of fruit to end your fast is papaya. The next best choices (in order of preference) are pear, peach, plum, apple, grapes, watermelon, or any fruit in season (no citrus). Be sure to eat only one fruit.

After eating the fruit, you will find that your taste buds have been aroused and you will probably feel like eating more. Don't! Don't try to satisfy your appetite with this meal; it won't work. After a cleansing program, the body assimilates food at a faster rate so you won't get that "filled up" feeling.

Lunch: Have your lunch in the early afternoon. Try a small mixed-green salad, such as lettuce (not iceberg), sprouts, tomatoes, celery, carrots, and cucumber. Don't use salad dressing and don't have a second helping. Squeeze a lemon on your salad if desired.

Dinner: Have another small vegetable salad or another fruit (do not mix fruit and vegetables). Try to eat this meal before 7:00 p.m.

Snacks: Have vegetable juice drinks, Bernard Jensen's Broth, or herbal teas in between meals if desired.

Second Day

You may begin any vitamin and mineral supplements you were taking prior to the cleansing program.

Breakfast: Fruit salad with or without yogurt (goat yogurt, preferably).

Lunch: Mixed vegetable salad; add some protein, such as avocado or tofu. A salad dressing is fine with this salad.

Dinner: Lightly steamed vegetables with brown rice or millet (moderate portions).

Third to Seventh Day

Continue eating salads, steamed vegetables, grains, fruits, and yogurt (goat preferred).

In the weeks following your cleansing, try cutting down on the size of your meals. Your body will feel better if you consume less food. Don't try to achieve the "filled up" feeling when eating. Don't eat late in the evening or, if you must, make it a light meal, such as a fruit salad.

Consider how much food you're eating and whether your food combinations are good. Continue to use the recommended products from your cleansing program (Pau D'Arco Tea, DDS Acidophilus, Bernard Jensen's Broth, fresh vegetable juices, and Whole Life Food Blend).

Repeat this cleansing program within three months.

5

Lactobacillus Acidophilus: The Well-Kept Secret

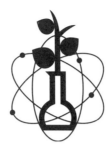

Lactobacillus Acidophilus: The Friendly Bacteria

Lactobacillus acidophilus is a healthful bacteria that lives in the colon. It inhibits the growth of disease-causing bacteria and is essential for normal digestion.

The routine use of antibiotics as medicine and the hidden consumption of antibiotics in meat, poultry, and dairy products destroys the natural, healthful bacteria your body needs to protect itself.

Every year in the United States over 35 million pounds of antibiotics are produced and their consumption is divided between livestock, poultry, and humans. Further, diets low in fiber and with few fresh, whole foods—and high in sugars, flours, fat, alcohol, or coffee—destroy *L. acidophilus* and encourage the growth of unfriendly putrefactive bacteria in the colon. This unfavorable shift in bacterial forms leaves you open to numerous kinds of infection and digestive distress.

L. acidophilus is a living food with unique health-giving properties. It has long been known to enhance digestion and nutrient absorption. It inhibits the growth of unfriendly bacteria, improves bowel regularity, and enhances natural immunity. *L. acidophilus* helps normalize blood cholesterol levels and even sweetens the breath.

Lactobacillus Acidophilus History

by Keith W. Sehnert, M.D.

Lactobacilli have been used in food preparation by nearly all of humankind. The Russians and Bulgarians prepared yogurt, the Danes and Germans made cheese, and the Japanese developed their miso.

In 1908, the Russian scientist Metchnikoff wrote that yogurt was the "elixir of life." He advanced the theory that yogurt could counteract the "putrefactive bacteria" in the large intestine that caused disease and shortened life. Metchnikoff reasoned that people in the Caucasus area around the Black Sea lived such long and healthy lives because of the great amount of Lactobacillus they ate in their food.

In 1986, the British nutritionist K. W. Heaton reported in the *Journal of the Royal Society of Medicine* about the Asian people from Gujarat. When these Indians, primarily of the Hindu faith, immigrate to London they develop a variety of nutritional problems. They have traditionally eaten kefir, a yogurt-like food fermented by Lactobacillus. Heaton also noted that in India they eat imperfectly washed vegetables that are likely covered with Lactobacillus from the soil in their gardens. When these people move to England, they eat well-washed British vegetables purchased from the local greengrocer. As time passes and the Indians become "more British" they begin eating an "endless variety of sugary foods and drinks," stop making kefir, and over a few years begin to "manifest a high prevalence of obesity, diabetes, and coronary heart disease."

A number of researchers over the years have reported on the complications resulting from the extensive use of antibiotics, emphasized the significance of a "bacterial equilibrium" in the intestinal tract, and observed the favorable influence of certain Lactobacilli in counteracting the overgrowth of pathogenic organisms in the intestinal flora. Digestive disorders, including diarrhea, constipation, irritable colon, and colitis, have been relieved by the administration of Lactobacillus. During 1950-60, some studies were conducted to compare *L. acidophilus* with neomycin sulfate to combat *E. coli* infection. *L. acidophilus* proved to be 97 percent as effective as neomycin sulfate in combating *E. coli* infection.

Lactobacillus Uses

During the nearly eight decades that marked the time between Metchnikoff and Heaton, much was learned about the Lactobacillus *family*. I emphasize the word "family" because the term "Lactobacillus" is a family name for a whole group of bacteria. They are described in bacteriology books as gram-positive, monmotile rods that ferment carbohydrates with the production of lactic acid and gas (mostly carbon dioxide). These are the bacteria that give the bubbles to champagne, the holes in Swiss cheese, and are the culprits that cause tooth decay.

Like persons with, for example, the family name of Smith, Lactobacilli have individual names and various jobs. The Smiths I know are Tom who is a banker and John who is a recreation director. The "clan" Lactobacillus has less common names and occupations. Casea makes cheese, Bulgaricus specializes in yogurt, and Fermentum turns grape juice into wine. There are many others, including the one we're interested in, acidophilus and its special strain, DDS.

Not All Lactobacilli Are the Same

Although the claims and labels may look the same for Lactobacillus products, the fact is they are not the same. As a result of my studies, I've decided to use DDS Acidophilus because of its stability, potency effectiveness, and lower cost.

Therapeutic Effects of DDS

Studies conducted by scientists at the University of Nebraska and Michigan State University have shown that DDS Acidophilus provides several therapeutic effects. It has specific actions including the ability to make a natural antibiotic, acidiophilin, and forms lactic acid and hydrogen peroxide.

Acidiophilin, the antibiotic, is active against a wide variety of gram-positive and gram-negative bacteria, such as *Streptococcus faecalis, Staphylococcus aureus,* and *Escherichea coli,* plus a host of others.

Acidophilin has also been found to retard the growth of *Candida albicans* in the laboratory. It should be noted that yogurt has long been used as a folk remedy for vaginitis. Lactobacillus organisms are normal constituents of vaginal flora. They contribute to the maintenance of the acid pH by fermenting glycogen in the mucous to lactic acid.

Nutritional Effects

In addition to the specific therapeutic effects of DDS, Lactobacilli in general help produce B vitamins (folic acid, niacin, riboflavin, B_{12}, B_6, and pantothenic acid); aid in predigestion of proteins and formation of free amino acids; help predigest lactose (which assists people with lactose intolerance due to lack of intestinal lactase and beta-galactosidase enzymes); and have anticholesteremic and antilipedemic effects.

Miscellaneous Actions

Epidemological studies show that the ingestion of cultured dairy products may reduce the risk of colon cancer. This action is thought to be due to the effects of *L. acidophilus* on fecal enzyme activity such as beta-glucuronidase and nitro-redyctase, which change procarcinogens (cancer causing chemicals) into less harmful substances.

Comparison of Commercial Products

After a review of the many Lactobacillus products, I agree with other experts that there are three criteria for consumers to consider:

1. Benefits associated with one particular strain may not necessarily apply to other strains of the same organism.
2. Commercial preparations shown to be effective in the laboratory may not contain sufficient numbers of living organisms to be of any clinical benefit.
3. Lactobacilli are fastidious in growth and metabolism, and are thus markedly affected by alcohol, antibiotic, and dietary components.

In an excellent review article, Hangee-Bauer noted that "Unfortunately, little data is available for comparing specific products, and many problems exist: many yogurts do not contain viable organisms (due to long shelf time and other factors) and products with even small amounts of glucose or sugar in them can inhibit the growth of Lactobacilli for as long as three days."

While University of Nebraska researchers and others have conducted extensive studies on DDS Acidophilus, U.A.S. Laboratories has developed unique manufacturing methods. These produce DDS on a rice starch base and avoid corn, soy, whey, lactose, and preservatives. U.A.S. has marketed this potent, stable, and effective strain since 1979. It is the most extensively researched commercial strain available.

Each DDS Acidophilus capsule contains more than one billion viable *L. acidophilus* organisms according to studies by a respected reference laboratory, A & L Midwest Agricultural Laboratories, 13611 "B" Street, Omaha, NE 68114.

General Summary of DDS Advantages

When the technical and research data on DDS were reviewed recently, these benefits were reported:

1. **Vitamin production:** DDS is capable of producing vitamins while many other Lactobacilli on the market require B vitamins for growth. The B-complex vitamins synthesized are niacin, pantothenic acid, pyrodoxine, biotin, B_6, B_{12}, and folic acid.
2. **Lactose intolerance:** Deficiency of lactase enzyme results in the inefficient digestion of lactose (milk sugar), a condition called lactose intolerance. DDS produces lactase enzyme, which helps digest lactose.
3. **Food digestion:** DDS produces enzymes that help digest food and decrease bloating.
4. **Reduces cholesterol:** DDS possesses anticholesteremic and antilipidemic factors. Several studies show significant reduction of serum cholesterol levels after supplementation with DDS.
5. **Prevents bad breath:** Colonization of putrefying bacteria in large numbers in the throat, tongue, and mouth causes halitosis (bad breath). When these putrefying bacteria are dominant in the intestine, they produce objectionable gases. DDS helps keep those putrefying bacteria in check, thus helping prevent bad breath.
6. **Natural antibiotic:** DDS is known to produce acidophilin, a natural antibiotic, which has been shown to possess (in vitro) a wide range of antimicrobial activity against common food-borne pathogens. The following organisms can be inhibited by acidophilin:
   Bacillus subtilis
   Bacillus cereus
   Bacillus stearothermophilus
   Streptococcus faecalis var. liquifaciens
   Streptococcus lactis
   Lactobacillus lactis
   Lactobacillus casei
   Lactobacillus plantarum
   Lactobacillus leichmannii

Sarcina lutea
Serratia marcescens
Proteus vulgaris
Escherichia coli
Salmonella typhosa
Salmonella schottmuelleri
Shigella dysenteriae
Shigella paradysenteriae
Pseudomonas fluorescens
Pseudomonas aeruginosa
Staphylococcus aureus
Klebsiella pneumoniae
Vibrio comma

7. **Antiviral effects:** *L. acidophilus* can inactivate many different viruses.

8. **Cold-sore management:** Cold sores (fever blisters) are caused by *Herpes simplex*, which often can be prevented or even cured by supplementation with DDS.

9. **Inhibition of Candida albicans:** Inhibition of this common yeast is possible with supplementation of DDS and this has been confirmed by clinical studies.

10. **Anticarcinogenic effects:** Studies at Sloan Kettering Institute for Cancer Research and the University of Nebraska show DDS to possess definite antitumor activity and to have inhibited tumor proliferation by 41 percent.

Conclusions

Persons who are heading to a health food store to buy a Lactobacillus product should remember the advice once given by a Roman philosopher: "caveat emptor" or "buyer beware." The labels and promotional literature of many products claim a high bacterial count only because they do not use pure *Lactobacillus acidophilus* and raise their count by using *other* bacteria in the mixture. Others have a low count on Lacto-bacillus organism because they were not properly stored after manufacturing was completed. Still others get around the truth by variations in dosage. Instead of the two capsules per day recommended for DDS, they advise "two to four capsules, two to four times per day," which is 16 capsules for a comparable dose! Other firms may promote their product by referring to DDS research—not their *own!* Ask the druggist or store manager to show you technical data on the product. Read it carefully. You will discover what I found: *not all Lactobacilli are the same!*

Reprinted by permission of Keith W. Sehnert, M.D.

Note: DDS Acidophilus has been developed in a rice starch base. No dairy, corn, soy, or preservatives have been added. It is also important to know that many acidophilus products do not colonize in the colon. DDS Acidophilus is acid-resistant and implants in the colon.

An order form for DDS Acidophilus capsules is on page 291.

Our Internal Microbial Community —Maintaining the Healthy Balance

by Nigel Plummer, Ph.D., Microbiology, University of Surrey, U.K.

It is true to say that we are largely unaware of the friendly microbial community which resides on our skin, and inside our respiratory, genito-urinary, and intestinal tracts. This is somewhat surprising given that they outnumber the total of our own tissue cells by 100:1, and make up about 50% of the weight of our feces. Moreover it should be noted that everything we ingest has to pass through the microbial community before we as the host assimilate it.

In general, the normal flora is very beneficial to our health, protecting us from infection by intestinal pathogens, enhancing the absorption of many nutrients, and detoxifying many of the pollutants we come into contact with on a daily basis. In addition to this there is recent scientific evidence that the normal flora is involved in reduction of cholesterol and the prevention of some forms of cancer.

Unfortunately, this delicate balance of the normal flora can be easily upset, and this can result from circumstances as varied as stressful lifestyle through to the use of prescription medicines. Indeed, probably the most common cause of severe disruption of the normal flora is the use of antibiotics.

Broad spectrum antibiotics are known to have a very major effect on both the numbers and types of the microbial population and one consequence of their use is that undesirable bacteria and yeasts often grow to replace the more beneficial types. These undesirable types can persist for months or years and can produce symptoms in the individual ranging from intermittant abdominal pain through diarrhea or constipation. These symptoms can become chronic and are very similar to those seen in Irritable Bowel Syndrome.

A unique new concept of microbial supplementation is now

available which tailors the treatment regime to the level of imbalance in the individual, with the result that in all cases the healthy flora is reestablished and then maintained at optimum levels for maximized long-term benefits. No other system or products differentiate the level of need in the individual and so very often have the effect dramatically under-supplying or over-supplying the beneficial bacteria.

The new system works at three levels:

1. Correcting Major Imbalance. This occurs most often following antibiotic therapy, and acute intestinal upset. Much of the normal flora is eradicated and needs to be replaced very rapidly if overgrowth is to be avoided. As such an intensive period of 14 days supplementation with very high numbers (30-50 billion/day) of beneficial bacteria is advised. After this the normal flora is well on the way to becoming established, and a more extended treatment is required to complete the process. This extended treatment is the same as would be advised for minor imbalance. The product used in this category is called **Replete**.

2. Correcting Minor Imbalance. This occurs in people who live with a stressful lifestyle, or who consume excessive alchohol, and also following general illness. To re-establish the correct microbial balance, a period of 6-8 weeks of an intermediate intensity of supplementation is required (4-5 billion/day). Following this period the flora will be in a balanced equilibrium, and the individual will be poised to obtain the long term benefits of this situation. However, this will only be insured if a maintenance level of beneifiial bacteria are supplemented on a daily basis to continually "top up" any sporadic instances of minor imbalance which may occur. The product used in this situation is called **HMF Forte**.

3. Maintaining the Healthy Balance. Once balance has been restored by the above regime, it needs to be maintained in order to achieve maximized benefits of the flora and also to help prevent the system giong out of balance again. By taking this level of beneficial bacteria (1 billion) on a daily basis—but only once the balance is already present—then a healthy beneficial flora is ensured. The product used for this is **HMF**.

Three Phase Intestinal Flora Rebuilding Program

Purpose: To prevent the overgrowth of undesirable bacterias and promote repopulation of beneficial bacteria and enhance removal and detoxification of residual antibodies. This Three Phase Program involves a systematic and *sequential use* of the following:

Level 1—Intensive. Product name: *Replete™ with FOS*

Daily dosage: $\frac{1}{2}$ - 1 envelope dissolved in water with a minimum of 30 billion viable microbes per day.

Duration: Every day for 7 - 14 days.

Strains: Strains of Bifidobacteria, Lactobacillus acidophilus and Lactobacillus brevis are administered. They all have the ability to colonize the gastrointestinal tract. Fructooligosaccharides (FOS) is used in conjunction with these cultures.

Benefits: Rapid establishment of the lactobacilli in the upper small intestine, with Bifidobacteria colonizing the ileum and the colon. Relief of abdominal complaints due to microflora imbalance. Crowding out of yeast and other undesirable bacteria.

Note: Replete should be ideally used the day the antibiotic course is over. If excessive gas develops during use of Replete, use $\frac{1}{2}$ envelope in the A.M. and $\frac{1}{2}$ in the P.M. Each envelope contains 30-40 billion organisms plus 13 grams Fructooligosaccharides (FOS).

Level 2—Follow On. Product name: *HMF Forte (in FOS base)*

Daily dosage: 1 capsule daily delivering a minimum total of 4 billion viable microbes.

Duration: Daily for 6 - 8 weeks.

Strains: High levels of L. acidophilus and Bifidobacteria with lower levels of Lactobacillus brevis. FOS is used in conjunction.

Benefits: Gradual shift of microbial population with beneficial bacteria becoming more dominant. Steady decrease in complaints due to minor imbalance in microflora. Completion of this stage should result in flora being healthy and "normal."

Note: The consumption of cooked oatmeal, fruits and vegetables rich in fermentable fiber (bananas, apples, yams, potatoes) provide excellent nourishment for promoting friendly bacteria growth.

Level 3— Maintenance. Product name: *HMF (in FOS base)*

Daily dosage: Minimum total of 1 billion viable microbes.

Duration: Continuous administration.

Strains: Equal numbers of L. acidophilus and Bifidobacteria in a vegetable FOS base.

Benefits: Continuous supplementation leads to long-term benefits of having optimized flora. Maintenance of healthy flora with lowered risk of imbalance occurring.

Additional Supplements

Before Breakfast:

1 teaspoon of *WheyPlex* - A concentrated fraction of whey that contains the nutrients that support our "gut" defenses.

With Breakfast:

1 capsule of *Poly VytaMyns* - Microcoated multiple vitamin-mineral formula with several cofactors.

1 capsule *Trival* - A 5000 year old formula with multiple distinct properties including a toning effect and gastrointestinal defense support.

1 tablet *Livit 2* - Standardized Ayurvedic botanical formula for liver support. Helps promote detoxification of residual antibiotics.

Before Lunch: 1 teaspoon *WheyPlex.*

With Lunch: 2 capsules *Poly VytaMyns*, 1 capsule *Trifal.*

Before Dinner: 1 teaspoon *WheyPlex*, 1 capsule *Trifal*

With Dinner: 2 tablets *Livit 2.*

To obtain the Three Phase Intestinal Rebuilding Program, please see the order form which begins on page 291.

6

Candida Albicans: The Quiet Epidemic

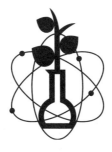

Candida Albicans Overgrowth

by William Wolcott

What is Candida?

Candida albicans is a yeast that lives in the mouth, throat, intestines, and genitourinary tract of most humans. Candida is usually considered to be a normal part of the bowel flora (the organisms that coexist in our lower digestive tract). A healthy immune system normally keeps candida under control, but when the immune system is weakened, the natural balance between the human host and the candida is altered. Unless the body's defenses are given some assistance, colonies of candida will flourish throughout the body producing many adverse physical and mental symptoms collectively known as candidiasis.

We all live in a virtual sea of microorganisms—bacteria, viruses, fungi, and so forth. These microbes can reside in the throat, mouth, nose, intestinal tract, or almost anywhere; they are as much a part of our bodies as the food we eat. Usually, these microorganisms do not cause illness, unless our resistance becomes lowered.

Candida is actually a member of a broader classification of organisms known as fungi. Traditionally, fungi are considered plants, but they contain no chlorophyll and cannot make their own food. Fungi are found in the air we breathe as well as in moist, shady soil, water, manure, dead leaves, fruit, leftover food, and in a wide variety of places and circumstances.

How Do You Get Candida?

Candida albicans prefers people. Candida enters newborn infants during or shortly after birth. Usually, the growth of the yeast is kept in check by the infant's immune system and thus produces no overt symptoms. But, should the immune response weaken, conditions known as oral thrush and diaper rash can result. By six months of age, 90 percent of all babies test positive for candida. And by adulthood, virtually all humans play host to *Candida albicans* and are thus engaged in a lifelong relationship.

Three primary factors weaken the immune system and promote the abnormal growth of candida in the body: 1) poor dietary habits, especially excessive intakes of sugars, starches, yeast-containing products, and processed food; 2) repeated use of antibiotics; 3) the use of hormonal medications such as corticosteroids and birth control pills; and 4) protozoa and other parasitic infestations.

Candida coexists in our bodies with many species of bacteria in a competitive balance. Other bacteria act in part to keep candida growth in check, unless that balance is upset. In a healthy person, the immune system keeps candida proliferation under control, but when the immune response is weakened, candida growth can proceed unhindered. Candida is an "opportunistic organism" which, when given the opportunity, will attempt to colonize all bodily tissues. The uncontrolled growth of candida is known as candida overgrowth.

Do You Have Candida?

- Do you have digestive problems such as indigestion, constipation, diarrhea, bloating, or gas?
- Have you, at any time in your life, taken antibiotics for acne, respiratory, urinary, or other infections?

- Have you taken corticosteroids or immunosuppressive drugs?
- Do you have a preference for sweets, breads, or alcoholic drinks?
- Are you bothered by athlete's foot, psoriasis, or other chronic fungal infestations of the skin?
- Have you ever been diagnosed with parasites?
- Have you ever been troubled with diarrhea or other intestinal problems when traveling?
- Do you experience fatigue, depression, poor memory, or nervous tension?
- Have you even been troubled by persistent prostatitis or vaginitis?
- Do you feel bad all over and no one has been able to determine why?

If you answered yes to three or more of the above questions, candida overgrowth may play a role in causing your symptoms.

Causes of Candida Overgrowth

It is well known that the immune system is highly dependent on the proper biochemical balance in the body. Unfortunately, there are many factors in our modern society that can upset the ecological balance of the body, weaken the immune system, and thus allow yeast to overgrow. Many physicians cognizant of candida report that 50 to 70 percent of their patients have candida overgrowth. These seemingly epidemic proportions are attributed to the general decline of vitality—specifically in relation to the immune system—in our society as a result of generations of suboptimal diets and other associated factors of drug and chemical exposure.

Traditional foods have been notably replaced by severely altered foods from a multitude of "modern" treatment methods in growing, processing, and packaging. Heating, pressurizing, preserving, refining, stabilizing, and even creating synthetic foods have all resulted in the considerable alteration of nutrient intake from what had been the previous norm for thousands of years.

Radical alterations in lifestyle that have accompanied rapid modernization in the twentieth century have brought unforseen and previously uncommon stresses that the human body must now cope with in its efforts at adaptation. Pollution of our air, water, and food; new medications and drugs, both prescription and nonprescription; alcohol; tobacco; high carbohydrate and sugar intake in our diets; chronic food and chemical allergies—all put a considerable strain on the immune system.

There is a growing awareness of the link between major illnesses, such as cancer, diabetes, heart disease, and schizophrenia, to diet and environmental factors and their adverse affects on the immune system. *Candida albicans,* usually a benign yeast held in check by the immune system, proliferates when the immune system becomes unbalanced, compromised, or weakened. The major risk factors that may predispose you to the proliferation of candida are the following:

Antibiotics and Sulfa Drugs. Probably the chief culprit of all, antibiotics kill all bacteria; they do not distinguish the good from the bad. Antibiotics kill the "good" flora that normally keep candida under control. This allows for unchecked growth of candida in the intestinal tract.

It is normally difficult to recover a yeast culture from bodily surfaces. However, after 48 hours of taking tetracycline, yeast can be cultivated easily from anyone. The prevalence today of candida may be most directly related to the widespread societal exposure to antibiotics—from prescriptions for colds, infections, and acne, and from the additional consumption of antibiotic-treated foods, such as meats, dairy, poultry, and eggs.

The rapid and direct proliferation of yeast following antibiotic use strongly suggests that the problem of candida is one that stems from an inner state of imbalance, rather than from an outside attack by a microbe or disease.

Steroid Hormones and Immunosuppressant Drugs. These drugs, such as cortisone, treat severe allergic problems by paralyzing the immune system's ability to react.

Pregnancy, Multiple Pregnancies, or Birth Control Pills. These upset the body's hormonal balance.

Improper Diet. Diets high in carbohydrates, sugar intake, yeast and yeast products, molds, and fermented foods encourage candida overgrowth.

Environmental Hazards. Prolonged exposure to environmental molds as well as an increasing number of chemicals in food, water, and air, including petrochemicals, formaldehyde, perfumes, cleaning fluids, insecticides, tobacco, and other indoor and outdoor pollutants, make the system more susceptible to yeast imbalance.

Once begun, candida overgrowth can result in a self-perpetuating, negative cycle if not recognized and treated appropriately. Large numbers of yeast colonies can weaken the immune system, which normally protects the body from harmful invaders. The immune system may concurrently be adversely affected by poor nutrition and heavy exposure to environmental toxins.

The resulting lowered resistance may not only cause an overall sense of ill health, or the development of respiratory, digestive, and other systemic symptoms. People may also become predisposed to developing sensitivities to foods and chemicals in the environment. Such "allergies" may in turn cause the membranes of the nose, throat, ears, bladder, and intestinal tract to swell and develop infection.

These conditions may lead the physician to prescribe a "broad spectrum" antibiotic that then further promotes the overgrowth of candida and strengthens the existing negative chain of events, leading to further stress on the immune system and increased candida-related problems.

What Are the Signs of Candida Infections?

The result of heightened candida overgrowth is a list of adverse symptoms of considerable length. Basically, the characteristics of candida overgrowth fall under three categories: those affecting the gastrointestinal and genitourinary tracts; allergic responses; and mental/emotional manifestations.

Initially, the signs will show near the sites of original yeast colonies. Most often, the first signs are seen in conditions such as nasal congestion and discharge, nasal itching, blisters in the mouth, sore or dry throat, abdominal pain, belching, bloating, heartburn, constipation, diarrhea, rectal burning or itching, vaginal discharge, vaginal itching or burning, increasingly worsening symptoms of PMS (premenstrual syndrome), prostatitis, impotence, frequent urination, burning on urination, and bladder infections.

But, if the immune system remains weak long enough, candida can spread to all parts of the body causing an additional plethora of problems. Most commonly these include the gastrointestinal tract with all manner of digestive disturbances, food allergies, sensitivities, and cravings for sweets; central nervous system disorders, such as fatigue, drowsiness, incoordination, lack of concentration, dizziness, headaches; musculoskeletal problems involving joint swelling, migrating aches and pains, and arthritis; hormonal disruptions, such as menstrual irregularities; problems with eyes, ears, and the respiratory system, such as spots in front of the eyes, failing vision, burning or tearing eyes, ear pain and deafness, bad breath, coughing, wheezing, asthma, and hay fever; skin problems, such as hives, rashes, eczema, psoriasis, dry skin, and chronic fungal infections, such as athlete's foot, ringworm, and fingernail/toenail infections; impairment of the circulatory system, such as cold hands and feet, numbness and tingling sensations; and aberrations in personality and behavior, such as anxiety, depression, hyperirritability, and mood swings.

In addition, 79 different toxic products are known to be

released by candida, which places a considerable burden on the immune system. These toxins get into the bloodstream and travel to all parts of the body where they may cause a host of adverse symptoms.

In candida overgrowth, the yeast colonies can dig deep into intestinal walls, damaging the bowel wall. Candida can also attack the immune system, causing supressor cell disease, in which the immune system produces antibodies to everything at the slightest provocation, resulting in extreme sensitivities. Finally, candida overgrowth can be dangerous if not controlled. The persistent, constant challenge to the immune system by an ever-increasing, long-term overgrowth of candida can eventually serve to wear down the immune system and cause a seriously weakened capacity for resistance to disease.

Women are more likely to get candida overgrowth than are men. This is related to the female sex hormone progesterone, which is elevated in the last half of the menstrual cycle. Progesterone increases the amount of glycogen (animal starch, easily converted to sugar) in the vaginal tissues, which provides an ideal growth medium for candida. Progesterone levels also elevate during pregnancy. Men are affected less frequently but are by no means invulnerable.

How Do You Know You Have Candida?

Currently, diagnosis is primarily clinical. Since almost all people have candida in their bodies, tests for its presence are useless; confirmation of overgrowth is very difficult through laboratory tests. And, since candida paralyzes the immune system, allergy tests to determine the system's reaction to it are also ineffectual.

Furthermore, the results of the yeast imbalance—the combined effects of different hormones, poisons generated and released by the yeast into the bloodstream, and the confusion created in the immune system—produce a wide variety of symptoms that are seemingly unrelated (such as wheezing, depression, and fungus infection under fingernails). Thus, it is difficult to make a definite diagnosis from any specific pattern of signs and symptoms.

Currently, the best test still seems to be the therapeutic trial. A joint decision is usually made by the physician and the patient after analyzing the individual's case history. (Many physicians regard vaginal yeast infections as the most reliable indicator of candida overgrowth in women, for example.) A tentative diagnosis is made, based on the patient's history of symptoms in relation to any known possible predisposing factors, which is then proven true or false by the way the patient responds to therapy.

Many physicians now believe that a clinical trial for candida overgrowth is of so little risk or expense that it should be considered in any chronic illness. One clinical trial you may try for five days is to avoid eating certain foods that are known to facilitate the growth of yeast. Such foods include the following:

Sugar and Carbohydrates found in all sweetened foods, including honey, molasses, sorghum, maple syrup, sugar, fructose, maltose, and dextrose. Also, fresh fruits, dried fruits, and fresh, frozen, and canned juices should be eliminated, as well as soda pop.

Yeast Products, such as beer, wine, sake, liquor, bread, natural B vitamins, and brewer's yeast.

Fermented and Mold Foods, such as mushrooms, cheese, vinegar, mustard, catsup, relish and other condiments made with vinegar, sour cream, buttermilk, tofu, soy sauce, and miso.

After eliminating these foods for five days, try adding them back into your diet in large quantities. By observing how you feel while off these foods, in comparison to any adverse affects experienced when going back on the foods, you may get a clue as to any possible yeast involvement as a causative factor for any adverse symptoms.

How Do You Reduce Candida Overgrowth?

Although diagnosis and supervision of treatment requires a physician, the reacquisition of health and control of candida by the immune system also depends a great deal on the effort of the candida patient. Generally, treatment of candida involves four major considerations:

1. Destroying the yeast.
2. Eliminating, if possible, immunosuppressive drugs and antibiotics, or curtailing their use to only when absolutely necessary.
3. Depriving the candida of those foods on which it is nourished and flourishes.
4. Rebalancing and strengthening of the body's immune system for the restoration of proper function through dietary measures that will meet individual nutritional requirements.

To destroy candida, or "to even the odds" so to speak, a physician may prescribe a drug by the name of nystatin, or one of several available products containing nystatin. It is an antibiotic, which means that it is made by one kind of germ, such as a mold, to kill another germ, such as strep, staph, or tuberculosis.

Nystatin is an antibiotic that kills yeasts and only yeasts. It is one of the least toxic known drugs; even when large amounts are ingested, only small traces actually get into the bloodstream. The pure powdered form is generally accepted as most effective.

Nystatin and caprylic acid products are deadly to candida. Depending on the severity of candida overgrowth and the amount of the agents taken, the candida can be killed off in vast numbers in a very short period of time. As they are killed, they release substances that are toxic to the body. If this process occurs more quickly than the toxins can be cleared from the bloodstream and eliminated by the body, a temporary toxic or allergic-type reaction can occur. The technical name for this experience is a "Herxheimer reaction," more commonly referred to as "die-off."

Usually die-off lasts only a few hours, although it can last several days. It can usually be controlled almost entirely by the amount of ingestion of the agent and the rate or frequency it is taken. Signs of Herxheimer reaction can be many and varied, but generally involve such discomfort as aching, bloating, nausea, and an overall "goopy sick" feeling, or a worsening of original symptoms. Fortunately, die-off is generally short in duration, and although uncomfortable, is at least a confirmation of the presence of candida and that something good is happening.

Exercise, colonics, and enemas are helpful in countering the adversities of die-off.

Although nystatin is very effective in killing candida, many people develop an allergic-type sensitivity to it with prolonged use. For this reason, many physicians are now considering alternatives for the job. Foremost among these is the use of products containing caprylic acid.

Caprylic acid is a natural substance, a fatty acid, that is totally lethal to candida. It is available over the counter and appears to be equal to nystatin in effectiveness, and is not known to produce the sensitivity side effects of nystatin. Of the caprylic acid products on the market, CAPRYSTATIN, KAPRY-CIDIN-A, and ORITHRUSH-D GARGLE, when used together, appear to be the most effective by virtue of their capacity to address the entire digestive tract.

Other natural aids in the fight against candida are garlic and Pau D'Arco (or Taheebo) tea, both believed to have natural fungicidal properties. Garlic is preferably taken raw, but may be effectively utilized in capsule form in a product called Arizona Natural Garlic.

Proper Diet

Research has found that the immune system is highly sensitive to the proper biochemical balance in the body, which affects the immune system's efficient functioning. A growing amount of nutritional research suggests that although everyone requires the same nutrients to maintain metabolic processes, different people need different amounts of nutrients to meet optimal requirements of their nutritional individuality.

For these reasons, HEALTHEXCEL provides a scientific means of identifying nutritional requirements based on the determination of the individual's "metabolic type," i.e., the genetically determined metabolic and nutritional parameters. It is because different people have different metabolic types, and therefore different needs for nutrition, that the allopathic, symptom-treatment approach in nutrition is baseless and so often ineffective. This further explains why, nutritionally, what helps make one person feel better may have little or no effect on another, or even make a third person feel worse. Once the metabolic type is determined, a diet and supplementation program can be recommended to meet individual nutrition requirements, thus providing an ideal means of restoring proper biochemical balance.

In addition, the use of natural, live acidophilus culture, such as that found in the product DDS, has been found helpful in aiding the body to restore the proper intestinal flora balance.

Many people with candida overgrowth find it very difficult to "get off" an antifungal agent, such as nystatin or caprylic acid, without a recurrence of the problem. In lieu of such circumstances, consider the following:

- If different people have different requirements for nutrition; and
- If the immune system is highly dependent on the proper biochemical balance to function efficiently; and
- If the immune system is supposed to keep candida in check; and
- If the problem of candida overgrowth recurs when you stop the antifungal agent, then it is possible that you are following a diet that is inappropriate for your immune system, which may in part be responsible for your body's failure to control the yeast.

Ideally, then, it is HEALTHEXCEL's recommendation that the attending physician suggest that anyone with candida overgrowth adhere to a diet that is correct for that person's metabolic type.

Unfortunately, it's not sufficient to get rid of the symptoms of candida overgrowth to the exclusion of the underlying cause of the problem—a compromised immune system. Thus, if you ignore your nutritional individuality, you may also find that although you are temporarily successful in ridding your system of candida, your success may be short-lived and you may experience a recurrence of the problem. The next logical step is to improve your overall immune efficiency by addressing your individual metabolic requirements.

Conclusion

Total elimination of yeast from the body is neither feasible nor desirable, considering that yeasts are very likely beneficial to the body when a proper balance exists. Treatment of candida overgrowth does not seek the eradication of candida from the person, but rather a *restoration of the proper and balanced relationship between the person and the yeast.*

Candida albicans, if uncontrolled, may indeed pose a serious threat to health and well-being. Another perspective, however, may view candida as a kind of "early warning system." Candida in a well-balanced body chemistry is merely a part of a greater environmental whole that provides some benefit to the host with whom it coexists.

It is only when the body chemistry becomes imbalanced and the immune system is compromised as a result that overgrowth becomes a problem to be reckoned with. It is a signal to us that drugs, improper foods, or other forms of distress have significantly weakened our defenses and undermined our good health. Viewed from this perspective, the presence of early warning signals afforded us by *Candida albicans* may actually allow for the avoidance of future disaster.

How to Fight Candida and Survive

by Tom Valentine

"Untreated systemic candidiasis has a mortality rate approaching 100 percent. Delay in treatment is dangerous and will almost certainly end in death of the patient."

That telling statement was written by Dr. Richard Hurley of London in a medical paper.

"When tests are done on estrogen levels, thyroid levels, or other hormone levels and people are suffering from these symptoms (candidiasis), the hormones are there in the bloodstream, but they are not activating any response."

Orian Truss, M.D., the leading authority on chronic candidiasis, made the statement above when describing the insidious attacks the common fungus *Candida albicans* makes on the human endocrine and immune systems.

Hormones are essential to our health, and our bloodstream must be literally crawling with them in order for our bodies to operate in a normal, balanced manner. When candidiasis takes hold of the endocrine system and imbalances hormonal function, a major health problem develops that has yet to be fully diagnosed and understood by the mainstream medical establishment.

Candidiasis has a way of disarming our immune systems, and if that sounds like AIDS (Acquired Immune Deficiency Syndrome) to you, join the club that is seeing more links between the two deadly infections than the establishment cares to admit.

There is strong sentiment among Americans that the drug-monopolized, bureaucratically-controlled medical establishment has failed them. More and more people are looking back at their medical histories and seeing that what they had previously suffered was undiagnosed chronic candidiasis.

A Natural War

There is a war going on inside every one of us. It's a war between natural microbes in our systems, and we have been losing for decades because of our medical establishment's combination of arrogance and ignorance, or criminal neglect, or both.

Our vital endocrine system (thyroid, thymus, parathyroid, pineal, pituitary, adrenal, pancreas, ovaries, testes) should not be infected by naturally occurring intestinal fungus. But, it is—with devastating, generally undiagnosed effects.

The drug industry lock on medical technology and education has helped create an arrogant ignorance within the profession that has been further enhanced by monopolistic bureaucracy. To now be told by courageous researchers, defying established dogma, that the "wonder drugs" of the past have unleashed an epidemic of immune-destroying chronic candidiasis, calls for charges of criminal negligence.

Why do a few independent researchers have to put their reputations on the line and "discover" that the common yeast, *Candida albicans*, is wreaking havoc with our national health? Why didn't the great institutions learn this natural fact decades ago? Hippocrates, the father of medicine, noted the common candida-caused infections of vaginitis and oral thrush more than 1,500 years before the microscope.

However, to point out the flaws and establish blame does not solve the problem. What's done is done. Now people must act to help themselves, and at the same time to force political changes that will result in a revamping of the medical bureaucracy.

The big problem is to stop candidiasis before it stops us. Candida has the upper hand because millions remain in ignorance and joyously starve their own systems while feeding the fungus.

AIDS—Plus

How bad is it? Let's look at the latest from the AIDS front.

Even those who don't know about candida have heard about AIDS. There's no link between the two, you say. One is virally caused, the other is a mold, you say.

Dr. Robert S. Mendelsohn has pointed out that a bulletin from the medical establishment (*FDA Drug Bulletin*) places some forms of candidiasis in a category now called "lesser AIDS."

In his February 1985 newsletter, the doctor who pointed out the flaws in his profession for the benefit of the people wrote:

The new, expanded definition of AIDS, of course, raises a new set of questions. The government doctors have reassured us that no cases of AIDS have been found in members of families of AIDS victims. However, with their new definition, those old studies become worthless until the families are restudied for these additional diseases.

Perhaps even more importantly, the HTLV-III test, like any other laboratory test, produces not only false-positive results, but false negatives. Therefore, if a person has one of these diseases now listed under the AIDS umbrella, how do the doctors know that, even in the absence of a positive AIDS blood test, the patient does not have AIDS?

In case you aren't confused enough , the *FDA Drug Bulletin* states: "In addition, idiopathic thrombocytopenia (a blood condition) is probably associated with the HTLV-III-III infection, as are a variety of non-life-threatening fungal and bacterial infectious processes..." The doctors call these manifestations lesser AIDS.

So now we have AIDS, ARC (AIDS related complex) and lesser AIDS. When it comes to the causes of AIDS or its symptomatology, do researchers or government doctors really know what they're talking about?

Based on the in-depth research of Dr. Orian Truss, a physician from Birmingham, Alabama, wrote *The Missing Diagnosis*, and is considered the world's top authority on chronic

candidiasis—which is much more than a simple yeast infection, even though the same critter is involved.

Dr. Truss has cured patients of debilitating conditions,
which had virtually wrecked their lives, by discovering that the
patients were not "neurotic," nor did they need "psychiatry"
simply because medicine could not correctly diagnose their
chronic candidiasis.

Candida Albicans

Candida albicans is among the most common yeasts,
molds, and fungi. It may be found in every human intestinal
tract from the mouth (it is especially fond of dentures) to the
anus, and in every vagina. Normally, the fungus is kept under
control by friendly bacteria, such as Lactobacillus acidophilus,
so it poses no threat to health.

Many times we hear a person say, "Oh, that's only a yeast
infection, that's not serious." This is an attitude nurtured by
the establishment's attitude. Obviously a wrong attitude.

"The yeast lives in everyone," Dr. Truss told *Acres U.S.A.*
"However, when it is stimulated by various factors, especially
antibiotics and birth control pills, it may establish a chronic
infection known as chronic candidiasis."

What happens, Dr. Truss explained, is that the yeast is not
affected by the broad spectrum antibiotics, which kill off the
friendly bacteria by the billions. Antibiotics are the worst, but
not the only, drug-induced cause for chronic candidiasis. With
the friendly bacteria obliterated, the fungus overgrows its nor-
malcy and the individual's immune system must deal with the
spreading mold. "Once candida gets into other tissues and
into the bloodstream, it has the ability to overcome the
immune system."

That sounds a lot like AIDS, does it not?

To make matters worse, researchers at the University of
Iowa discovered that *Candida albicans* has chameleon-like
abilities to change its form—making it difficult to control.

According to the *Des Moines Register*, December 30, 1985, biologists at the University of Iowa described the common fungus as "a microscopic monster capable of inflicting a wide range of torture" on patients. "Until recently, however, nobody knew candida very well. Now it appears the common yeast is a more terrible creature than anyone suspected—a Dr. Jekyll and Mr. Hyde character capable of changing back to its original form."

Another aspect that sounds like AIDS!

"Dr. David Soll, the University of Iowa biologist who discovered candida's quick-change ability, says it may be what allows the fungus to elude both antibiotics and the body's immune system," the article added.

It is incredible that the wonders of modern medical technology somehow overlooked this fungus until Dr. Truss and others screamed so loudly they could no longer be ignored.

Now, we note, a number of financial grants are finding their way into universities as the drug monopoly scurries to cover its proverbial behind with patentable pharmacology to stop the spread of this common critter that drugs helped unleash in the first place.

In our technological sophistication, arrogant mankind seems to forget that "it isn't wise to fool mother nature."

Among the data from the study was the discovery that a particular drug, ketoconazole, does not work for "immunosuppressed patients." Immunosuppression is curious logic, unless you think you're smarter than nature.

According to Dr. Truss:

An immunosuppressant drug is a drug that suppresses or weakens the immune defenses of the body. Many symptoms of illness are actually due to the inflammation that results when the white blood cells respond in defense against some injurious or potentially dangerous factor.

Symptoms may be due to the body's defensive response to a germ, rather than to the germ itself. A sore throat or the inflamed tissues of the nose and throat characteristic of the common cold are familiar examples. Even when the inflammation is not clearly related to an infectious agent, for example rheumatoid arthritis, it is quite likely that most of the symptoms result from the immune response to an as yet undiscovered cause of the disease.

Since inflammation is distressing to patients, the medical profession happily accepted from drug manufacturers a group of drugs designed to suppress the immune system and make the inflammation go away.

"Unfortunately," Dr. Truss added, "it is not possible to suppress just one manifestation of immunity by impairing the entire immune response."

Cortisone-type hormone drugs are the most commonly used immunosuppressants, and Dr. Truss lists them among the major causes of the epidemic spread of chronic candidiasis.

Contributing Factors

Let's add it all up. Our society is crawling with pollutants that enhance candida and clobber us. Our food is refined, additivized, and chemicalized, and then so loaded with sugars and starch that we feed candida very happily—beer-belly bloat is an obvious "sign" of candidiasis.

There is also the "health food" known as brewer's yeast. Most B vitamins come in brewer's yeast bases, which serves to strengthen candida.

Infants being breastfed, Dr. Truss said, have a strong *Lactobacillus acidophilus* count and candidiasis is not normally seen. But once off the breast, candidiasis shows up in a hurry—as diaper rash.

The critter is chasing us from cradle to grave—gleefully. One doctor noted that "the living human is nothing more than organic matter that needs recycling to *Candida albicans.*"

Antibiotics are everywhere in our society—in meats and

poultry, in the hands of every pediatrician, even over-the-counter. Add the technical wonders of cortisone and birth control pills and you have an epidemic.

The symptoms of chronic candidiasis include:

Central nervous system disorders: depression, anxiety, irrational irritability, lethargy, fatigue, agitation, inability to concentrate, memory loss, and headaches, including migraines.

Intestinal disorders: bloating, diarrhea, constipation, heartburn, gastritis, indigestion, and colitis.

Allergic manifestations: severe chemical and food sensitivities, asthma, acne, hives, sinusitis, hay fever, skin rashes, earaches, and possible psoriasis.

In children there are hyperactivity, irritability, learning problems, poor appetite, and erratic sleep patterns as well as the other symptoms. One of the most used, if not the most used, medical techniques today is the ear-tube operation for children.

What can you do to protect yourself?

Doctors are prescribing nystatin and other prescription drugs, but as with all drugs there are drawbacks and side effects. Besides, there is evidence that when the drugs are halted, the yeast comes back with a vengeance. Some herbalists suggest garlic, but doctors say it is ineffective.

There are a number of independent physicians striving to cope with the pandemic, which is still largely unrecognized by the medical establishment. The best way to avoid or overcome chronic candidiasis is by following a careful dietary program, re-establishing the friendly bacteria, and strengthening the immune system.

Nothing fights *Candida albicans*, in all its forms, better than *Lactobacillus acidophilus*, especially the DDS strain developed at the University of Nebraska.

Note: There is an order form for the *Healing Within* Candida Overgrowth Elimination Program beginning on page 291. This time-proven program is highly effective in combating candida.

Candida Albicans Self-Test

Introduction

The following questionnaire was designed by William G. Crook, M.D., to be used by adults to identify their predisposition to *Candida albicans* yeast infection. It is not intended as a means for diagnosis, but only as an organized system for gathering information regarding candida. If you score high on this questionnaire, you may wish to bring it to your physician's attention. Your physician may then decide to run clinical tests in order to determine whether or not you have abnormal candida growth presently occurring. Any therapy in this regard will depend on your physician's judgment.

It is not within the jurisdiction of the author to diagnose the presence of candida, nor to recommend any therapeutic action. The author recognizes this activity as the sole responsibility of the attending physician. This material is provided for educational and informational purposes only, in hopes that it may prove of use to you and your physician.

Instructions

Section A pertains to factors in your medical history that may promote the imbalanced growth of candida. Sections B and C are concerned with symptoms commonly seen in individuals with yeast-connected illnesses.

For each "Yes" answer you have in Section A, circle the Point Score in that section. At the end of the section, total your score and record it on the Total Score line. Then move to Sections B and C, and score as indicated.

Section A: History

	Point Score
Have you taken tetracyclines (Sumycin®, Panmycin®, Vibramycin®, Minocin®, etc.) or other antibiotics for acne for one month or longer?	25
Have you at any time in your life taken other "broad-spectrum" antibiotics (ampicillin, amoxicillin, Ceclor®, Bactrim®, Septra®, Keflex®, etc.) for respiratory, urinary, or other infections for two months or longer, or in shorter course, four or more times in a one-year period?	20
Have you taken a broad-spectrum antibiotic drug, even a single course?	6
Have you at any time in your life been bothered by persistent prostatitis, vaginitis, or other problems affecting your reproductive organs?	25

Have you been pregnant:
Two or more times?	5
One time?	3

Have you taken birth control pills:
For more than two years?	15
For two weeks or less?	8

Have you taken prednisone, Decadron®, or other cortisone-type drugs:
For more than two weeks?	15
For two weeks or less?	6

	Point Score
Have you ever been afflicted with a parasitic problem at any time in your life?	20
Does exposure to perfumes, insecticides, fabric shop odors, and other chemicals provoke:	
Moderate or severe symptoms?	20
Mild symptoms?	5
Are symptoms worse on damp, muggy days or in moldy places?	20
Have you had athlete's foot, ringworm, jock itch, or other chronic fungus infections of the skin or nails:	
Severe or persistent?	20
Mild to moderate?	10
Do you crave sugar?	10
Do you crave breads?	10
Do you crave alcoholic beverages?	10
Does tobacco smoke really bother you?	10
Total Score Section A	_____

Section B: Major Symptoms

For each of your symptoms, enter the appropriate figure in the
Point Score column:
If a symptom is *occasional or mild*, score 3 points.
If a symptom is *frequent and/or moderately severe*, score 6 points.
If a symptom is *severe and/or disabling*, score 9 points.

	Point Score
Fatigue or lethargy	_____
Feeling of being drained	_____
Poor memory	_____
Feeling spacey or unreal	_____
Depression	_____
Numbness, burning, or tingling	_____
Muscle aches	_____
Muscle weakness or paralysis	_____
Pain and/or swelling in joints	_____
Abdominal pain	_____
Constipation	_____
Diarrhea	_____
Bloating	_____

Point Score

Troublesome vaginal discharge   _____

Persistent vaginal burning or itching   _____

Prostatitis   _____

Impotence   _____

Loss of sexual desire   _____

Endometriosis   _____

Cramps and/or other menstrual irregularities   _____

Premenstrual tension (PMS)   _____

Spots in front of eyes   _____

Erratic vision   _____

Total Score Section B   _____

Section C: Other Symptoms

For each of your symptoms, enter the appropriate figure in the Point Score column:
If a symptom is *occasional or mild*, score 3 points.
If a symptom is *frequent and/or moderately severe*, score 6 points.
If a symptom is *severe and/or disabling*, score 9 points.

	Point Score
Drowsiness	_____
Irritability or jitteriness	_____
Incoordination	_____
Inability to concentrate	_____
Frequent mood swings	_____
Headaches	_____
Dizziness/loss of balance	_____
Pressure above ears; feeling of head swelling or tingling	_____
Itching	_____
Other rashes	_____
Heartburn	_____
Indigestion	_____
Belching and intestinal gas	_____
Mucous in stools	_____
Hemorrhoids	_____
Dry mouth	_____

Point Score

Rash or blisters in mouth	_____
Bad breath	_____
Joint swelling or arthritis	_____
Nasal congestion or discharge	_____
Postnasal drip	_____
Nasal twitching	_____
Sore or dry throat	_____
Cough	_____
Pain or tightness in chest	_____
Wheezing or shortness of breath	_____
Urgency or urinary frequency	_____
Burning on urination	_____
Failing vision	_____
Burning or tearing of eyes	_____
Recurrent infections or fluid in ears	_____
Ear pain or deafness	_____
Total Score Section C	_____
Total Score Section A (from page 23)	_____
Total Score Section B (from page 25)	_____
Grand Total Score	_____

Scoring

According to Dr. Crook, yeast-connected health problems are *almost certainly* present in women with scores over 180, and in men with scores over 140. (Women's scores will tend to run higher, as seven items apply exclusively to women, while only two apply exclusively to men.)

Yeast-connected health problems are *probably* present in women with scores over 120, and in men with scores over 90.

Yeast-connected health problems are *possibly* present in women with scores over 60, and in men with scores over 40.

If you feel that you may have a candida overgrowth problem, consider following the *Healing Within* 8-Week Candida Overgrowth Elimination Program described on pages 167-178.

Oxygen Therapy

Why It Should Be of Interest to Everyone

For many years the health sciences have been seeking to identify the primary physical cause of all illness and disease, and create a universal remedy that would satisfy the correction of this primary cause. Now both have been found, but their utter simplicity makes them difficult to accept at first.

A toxic digestive system, organ system, and cellular environment is the primary cause of all ailments according to natural principles—not microbes, as we have been led to believe. No one should judge his or her health on the basis of daily evacuations of kidneys or bowels. A person may have regular daily "normal" eliminations, yet still be badly ailing because the assimilation and elimination processes may be unbalanced.

Oxygen Therapy accomplishes the necessary and desired purification of the digestive tract, then purifies every organ, blood vessel, and cell in the entire body. It does this not by burying symptoms as in drug therapy, but by liquefying the waste in the system and passing it out through the bowels and urinary tract.

Growing in the toxic (anaerobic) cellular environment are the microbes (bacteria, viruses, yeast, parasites, etc.) that we hear about so often in medical diagnosis as the main cause of illness or disease. These microbes cannot live in an oxygen-filled (aerobic) environment. You might notice here that Oxygen Therapy not only oxidizes the microbes, thus killing them off, but also eliminates the root cause of their presence in the first place—toxicity in the system.

Oxygen Therapy is an important natural nutritional method for the prevention and elimination of illness and disease. It can be used without interruption of one's work or activities.

Nature demands her time and cannot be hurried. Mild cases of ailments or illness may show splendid results in a few days or weeks, while in more serious cases a marked improvement cannot be expected in so short a time. Nevertheless, the longer the remedy is taken, the more marked the improvement. In more chronic or stubborn so-called incurable diseases, it should not be overlooked that the built-up toxins and medical poisons used to bury symptoms have impaired the metabolism, and cannot be rectified quickly, even by the best of healing methods. Because Oxygen Therapy employs nature's best natural resources and nothing else, its consistent use will not harm, but will give the best possible results.

At the start of Oxygen Therapy, the frequent watery stools, which may appear 3-5 times a day, will cease as soon as your body's system is purified. After that, you may increase your dose if so desired. The released oxygen will follow the blood stream, cleansing the blood vessels and cells. This being the case, we must allow time for the oxygen to reach the extreme parts of the body. Thus, it is impossible to gauge the exact time required for the correction of each case.

The results do not depend on dietary rules, but, of course, far better results are obtained if you refrain from consuming food or drink detrimental to your health. Even a person adhering to an unbalanced diet will feel beneficial results if general rules are consistently followed.

A healing process or reaction (sometimes called a healing crisis) may appear in many cases soon after starting Oxygen Therapy and may reappear at certain intervals in all ailments, especially chronic conditions, until the cause or causes of the ailments are eliminated. This healing process is an act of health which is naturally and nutritionally sound, and no one should become alarmed or discouraged through these natural healing reactions. On the contrary, they should be considered highly welcome as the true signs of a better and healthier future.

Summary

1. A toxic body has to be purified.
2. The damages done by ailments, disease or stress must be repaired.
3. An unhealthy metabolism must be balanced.

These three processes are required to return the body to complete health. Oxygen Therapy goes a long way toward satisfying these requirements for good health. Thousands of people are discovering Oxygen Therapy to be safe and effective against an amazing variety of disorders.

Dr. Joseph LaVolpa, N.D., P.M.D., Ph.D.
Preventive Medicine Specialist
Natural Health Center
Santa Rosa, California

Dear Friends in Health,

What I have to share with you is of such importance that I strongly encourage you to please read through this letter carefully.

Are you experiencing aging problems, lack of energy, ailments, or any kind of physical disorder that is preventing you from enjoying life? Have you tried everything available on the market and given up finding a cure? Please don't despair. There is something you can do, but you may not have heard about it until NOW. I'm talking about OXYGEN THERAPY, and it is available now for the first time in a stabilized powder in capsule form for convenient daily use.

Why oxygen? Here in the 1990s, we are taking in one-half the amount of oxygen of 100 years ago. Since we are an oxygen machine, this lack of oxygen means a significant reduction in our ability to recreate healthy cells.

It also means we are creating an internal environment designed for the growth of all kinds of bacteria, viruses, yeasts and toxins. These microbes and toxins cannot exist in an oxygen-filled environment.

It is for this reason that Oxygen Therapy is a breakthrough of staggering and immense importance.

Oxygen Therapy has demonstrated to be a powerful and effective remedy for:

AIDS	*Flu*
Allergies	*Hepatitis*
Arthritis	*Herpes*
Asthma	*HIV*
Cancer	*Metabolic Disorders*
Candida Yeast Infection	*Parasites*
Chronic Fatigue	*Reproductive Problems*
Circulatory Congestion	*Skin Eruptions*
Diabetes	*Tumors*
Digestive Disorders	*Urinary Disorders*
Epstein-Barr	

I give Oxygen Therapy my strongest endorsement. As a natural doctor, I believe in its capabilities. I know that it works because I've used it with my clients/patients and they report excellent results.

Be young again and live an active physical life free from disease and physical limitation. For the sake of your health and the health of your family, I urge you to try Oxygen Therapy today.

With healthy regards,

Dr. Joseph LaVolpa

Ozone: Its Therapeutic Action

Ozone (O_3 or O_2O) is an allotropic form of oxygen. It is oxygen in its most active state. It therefore means a more generous supply of oxygen, the life giver and life sustainer.

Through the action of flashes of lightning, nature produces Ozone to purify the air and to destroy all organic decay upon which disease, germs, and bacteria thrive. Like oxygen, Ozone is a healthful gas. It has, however, a much greater oxidizing, antiseptic, and germicidal power, and for this reason it is used with great success for the relief of various diseases. Recently, the FDA and other such suppressive organizations have been trying to negate the beneficial and life-sustaining qualities of Ozone by telling the public that Ozone is poisonous and detrimental to the body. This is not so! For years physicians around the world have used Ozone to bring palliative and curative results to many, many individuals. Famous physicians like Dr. Rokitansky in Vienna, Dr. F. M. Eugene Blass, and others around the world have realized the importance of this tremendous gas.

Ozone is one of the most energetic and useful agents known to science. Its therapeutic action is due to the oxygenation of the blood by the loose molecule (free radical) of oxygen in the O_3 compound. Ozone is carried to the various organs and tissues of the body and absorbed, thus oxidizing waste products and facilitating their elimination. In other words, Ozone increases the metabolism without the expenditure of vital energy. Special stress should be laid on the fact that Ozone is a *natural* remedy.

In the process of respiration, waste products are exposed to the action of the oxygen of the air, and they are burned up very much as if they were put into a stove, thereby producing body heat. In the living body, heat—whether tangible or not—is continually being generated through the chemical action of carbon and oxygen.

When the blood receives sufficient oxygen to unite with carbon, in the proportion of two atoms of oxygen to one of carbon, carbon dioxide or carbonic acid gas (CO_2) is formed, which is in a suitable state to be eliminated. The process of oxidation is complete, the body temperature is maintained at normal (98.6° F), the organs perform their functions properly, and the system is in a condition to resist the toxic influences of microbes, the environment, and mankind's excesses.

When, however, an insufficient amount of oxygen is received by the blood, carbon monoxide is formed (CO), which is not readily eliminated. Through its poisonous irritation to the organs, the body temperature is reduced below normal. The system is rendered incapable of resisting the toxic influences of the various bacteria, environmental and industrial-related toxins—disease is the result.

So prevalent is subnormal temperature among people who are "rundown," that nine out of ten of them show a subnormal temperature by actual thermometer test. There have been several reasons for subnormal temperatures in recent years. They range from "thyroid insufficiency" to "hypothalamus disorders." These explanations are correct—but only to a degree. The real *cause* of the problem is low and inadequate oxidation or oxygen assimilation. Therefore, the thyroid, hypothalamus, or other endocrine organs (given as the cause) are hindered in their normal metabolic functions, and subnormal temperature is the result. The correct way to counteract this situation is to give a substance that will restore the oxidative process.

The clinical thermometer is the best means of determining the existence of under-oxidation and should be used routinely. The temperature of a person who is under-oxidized runs from a fraction to several degrees below normal.

The under-oxidated and subnormal temperatured person will present one or more of the following symptoms: headache, dizziness, insomnia, constipation, feeling faint, loss of appetite, palpitation of the heart, bad kidney action, sporadic and related menstrual problems, cold hands and feet, and various other symptoms, all of which are due to an impoverished blood supply.

From these symptoms, we are justified in rendering an explanation of under-oxidation, taking on the definite form(s) of neurasthenia, liver disorders, kidney disorders, stomach and intestinal troubles, female disorders, melancholia, hysteria, chorea, anemia, chlorosis, sexual disorders, and so forth.

The symptoms or conditions that arise from a subnormal temperature are not necessarily in proportion to the degree of subnormal temperature. A person showing a fractional part of one degree of subnormal temperature may present problems or conditions of disease as severe as a person whose temperature is several degrees below normal.

A sufficiency of an active form of oxygen for the blood means better blood, better circulation, better assimilation, better equilibrium of body temperature, better vasomotor activity, better digestion, better elimination of waste products, less chance of auto-intoxication or toxemia (which is the keynote of many diseases), better chance for body building natural substances, and less chance of infection and disease.

After careful analytical investigation of disease, it has been demonstrated:

First: That one of the most common and important conditions that the person is called upon to correct is the weakness and incapacity produced by an impoverished or diminished blood supply.

Second: That under-oxidation produces bad health primarily because of an insufficient supply of oxygen; guaranteeing the formation of carbon monoxide, which is at once a de-oxidizer, hemoglobin destroyer, and irritant poison devitalizing the blood and paving the way to a multiplicity of acute troubles, many of which become chronic.

It has long been recognized that the atmosphere possesses the properties of blood-building, oxidation, and antisepsis.

Ozone differs from atmospheric action only in degree of activity and potency. Ozone's activity makes it the greatest blood building, oxidizing, and antiseptic agent within the reach of mankind.

It has been suggested that a subnormal temperature may be a normal condition with some people. This deduction can be disproven by placing anyone with a subnormal temperature under the active influence of Ozone and having the temperature rise back to normal.

Almost all forms of nervous, functional, respiratory, and blood disorders can be successfully corrected by oxidation restoration. The effects are perfectly natural, the nerves being left calm and toned with a feeling of buoyancy and exhilaration. Oxygen restoration stimulates the vasomotor system through the nerve centers, demonstrated by increased redness of the skin, a feeling of warmth throughout the whole body, and freer elimination of waste products. The Ozone treatment shows that poor oxidation is the cause of many disorders, by reason of the fact that when the temperature is brought up to normal, problems disappear.

Oxidation is the source of life!!!

—International Oxidation Institute, ASMM

7

Products for Candida Control

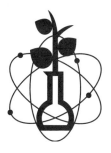

Oxy-Oxc

The Next Generation in Superoxygenation

Most people's primary nutritional focus is on the food and liquids they orally ingest. We take for granted that the nutrient given the highest priority by the body is oxygen, the lack of which will kill a human in a matter of minutes. Our planetary oxygen supply is becoming increasingly more toxic and its supply decreased by man-made pollutants. It is obvious that the oxygen we inhale has been greatly contaminated, especially in the inner cities. Therefore, it makes sense that enhancing one's cellular storehouse of oxygen can offset these ever-worsening conditions.

In his 1966 speech, "The Prime Cause and Prevention of Cancer," presented at the annual meeting of Nobelists in Lindau, Germany, Dr. Otto Warburg states:

Cancer, above all other diseases, has countless secondary causes. Almost anything can cause cancer but, even for cancer, there is only one prime cause. Summarized in a few words, the prime cause of cancer is the replacement of the respiration of oxygen in normal cells by a fermentation of sugar. All normal cells meet their energy needs by respiration of oxygen, whereas cancer cells meet their energy needs in great part by fermentation. All normal cells are thus obligate aerobes, whereas all cancer cells are partial anaerobes. From the standpoint of the physics and chemistry of life, this difference between normal and cancer cells is so great that one can scarcely picture a greater difference. Oxygen gas, the donor of energy in plants and animals, is dethroned in the cancer cells and replaced by an energy-yielding reaction of the lowest living forms.

A cell cannot become cancerous if its respiration is intact. Three ways are known to maintain a cell's respiration:
1. Add active groups of respiratory enzymes to your foods;
2. Saturate all growing body cells with oxygen; and
3. Keep away from external carcinogens.

Everyone knows we cannot live long without oxygen. However, many of us may be victims of a "low oxygen" condition caused by poor food, lack of exercise, polluted air, and shallow breathing. If our metabolism is not allowed to process food at the highest level of energy (high oxygen environment), our cells begin to accumulate waste products faster than the body can remove them, which in turn attracts harmful viruses and microbes (such as in flu, colds, toxic colon conditions, arterial plaque, cancer, and AIDS). If, however, the oxygen level around these anaerobic life forms is increased, they die! This may sound too simple, but there have been over 5,000 articles available in medical journals in the past 20 years regarding the action of oxygen products on pathogens.

Now you will be able to experience and benefit from Nature's simple yet powerful "product"—oxygen.

Oxy-Oxc (pronounced "OX-ee-OX-ee") is an evolutionary breakthrough in oxygen nutrition. Through an advanced proprietary process, triatomic oxygen (Ozone) is bonded through a crystal lattice matrix with magnesium peroxide, allowing a multifaceted approach to cellular oxygenation.

What Are the Contents of Oxy-Oxc?

A specially formulated Magnesium Peroxide Compound with Ozone/Oxygen enhancement and Vitamin C with a Bioflavonoid Complex.

What Does Oxy-Oxc Do?

It is a body oxygenator and energizer which detoxifies and cleanses wastes, pathogens, and plaque from the gastro-intestinal tract, colon, arteries, blood, etc.

Why Is Oxy-Oxc Needed?

As a result of poor diet, lack of exercise, polluted air, shallow breathing, and stress, many of us are in a low oxygen/toxic state. This creates inefficient metabolism, causing the body to accumulate waste products faster than it can eliminate them. This then leads to a favorable environment for the proliferation of pathogenic microbes (viruses, bacteria, fungi, etc.) which, in turn, create disease conditions (flu, herpes, candida, chronic fatigue, cancer, AIDS, etc.) If, however, the oxygen level around these anaerobic pathogens is increased, they die, unable to survive the high-oxygen environment.

How Does Oxy-Oxc Work?

As Oxy-Oxc reaches the stomach's acid environment and continues into the bloodstream, the Vitamin C (ascorbic acid) and bioflavonoid complex break the magnesium peroxide bond, releasing the Ozone and peroxides, softening the intestinal and arterial plaque, and killing pathogenic microbes throughout the body. The Ozone and peroxides further break down into oxygen which continues to purify and energize all cells in the body. As the liquefied plaques and dead pathogens move toward leaving the body, the magnesium creates a colon flushing reaction, increasing bowel activity and preventing reabsorption of the toxins.

How Is Oxy-Oxc Made?

Through an advanced proprietary process, Ozone, peroxides, and magnesium are merged and bonded into a crystal lattice matrix (similar to air bubbles in ice). Vitamin C and a whole-fruit bioflavonoid complex are added to help break the bond and provide a more sustained release, thus creating optimal assimilation.

Pau D'Arco Tea and Colon 8 Intestinal Cleanser

Pau D'Arco tea is made from tree bark imported from South America, where it has been in use for centuries. It has only recently received recognition in this country as a powerful healing tea and safe, natural antibiotic. It is very effective in reducing congestion throughout the lymph system as well as the lungs. It also helps clear mucous and acid buildup in the body. Pau D'Arco tea is a powerful aid for the immune system and the elimination of candida overgrowth.

Instructions: Add 1 heaping tablespoon of Pau D'Arco tea bark to 1 quart of water. Bring to a boil, then simmer for 20 minutes. Strain off the bark, allow the tea to cool, and refrigerate. Drink no more than 8 ounces daily, hot or cold. Continue to drink this tea after completing the candida reduction program; make it a regular part of your diet.

Colon 8 Intestinal Cleanser

Colon 8 Intestinal Cleanser is a mixture of herbs that scrubs and cleanses both the small intestine and the colon (large intestine). It will remove buildup of undigested food and mucous that may be lining the digestive and elimination system. Colon 8 is all natural and contains psyllium in a base of bentonite, oat bran, *Lactobacillus acidophilus*, whey, alfalfa, rhubarb, buckthorn, golden seal, gentian, cascara sagrada, aloe socotrina, calcium, magnesium, and other minerals natural to the herbs. This product contains no preservatives, salt, or artificial colors.

DDS Acidophilus Culture

DDS Acidophilus culture is one of just a few brands of acidophilus that is acid resistant and can survive the long journey through the digestive tract to the colon. DDS delivers one billion friendly bacteria in each capsule. These bacteria will colonize and re-establish the much needed friendly flora that may be absent due to past antibiotic use. DDS helps improve bowel movements and has an excellent cleansing effect on the liver. Acidophilus is also known to reduce blood cholesterol levels.

DDS should be taken with water only, first thing in the morning. DDS should not be taken with food or other liquids because these substances stimulate the natural stomach acids, weakening the ability of DDS to recolonize in the colon.

Not All Lactobacilli Are the Same

Although the claims and labels may look the same for Lactobacillus products, the fact is they are not the same. As a result of my studies, I've decided to use DDS Acidophilus because of its stability, potency effectiveness, and lower cost.

Therapeutic Effects of DDS

Studies conducted by scientists at the University of Nebraska and Michigan State University have shown that DDS Acidophilus provides several therapeutic effects. Its specific actions include the ability to make a natural antibiotic, acidiophilin, and form lactic acid and hydrogen peroxide.

Acidiophilin, the antibiotic, is active against a wide variety of gram-positive and gram-negative bacteria, such as Streptococcus faecalis, Staphylococcus aureus, and Escherichea coli, plus a host of others.

Acidophilin has also been found to retard the growth of *Candida albicans* in the laboratory. It should be noted that yogurt has long been used as a folk remedy for vaginitis. Lactobacillus organisms are normal constituents of vaginal flora. They contribute to the maintenance of the acid pH by fermenting glycogen in the mucous to lactic acid.

Nutritional Effects

In addition to the specific therapeutic effects of DDS, Lactobacilli in general help produce B vitamins (folic acid, niacin, riboflavin, B_{12}, B_6, and pantothenic acid); aid in predigestion of proteins and formation of free amino acids; help predigest lactose (which assists people with lactose intolerance due to lack of intestinal lactase and beta-galactosidase enzymes); and have anticholesteremic and antilipedemic effects.

CHAPTER 7

Caprystatin, Kaprycidin-A
and Orithrush-D

Caprystatin contains reagent-grade caprylic acid (100 mg.) adsorbed to a non-resinous anion-exchange moiety to provide prolonged release throughout the surface area of the lower bowel. Caprystatin contains no phenols, formaldehyde, resins, or other commonly reactive ingredients. It is an effective agent to help reduce candida overgrowth in the colon.

Kaprycidin-A

Kaprycidin-A contains an encapsulated form of caprylic acid (325 mg.) as calcium, magnesium, and zinc caprylates. This time-delayed caprylate complex is designed for smooth release through the gastrointestinal tract. It may be used together with Caprystatin to reduce candida overgrowth throughout the intestinal tract. Kaprycidin-A's primary action is in the small intestine.

Orithrush-D

This formula includes a specially buffered solution of sorbic acid. When diluted one part Orithrush-D to 20 parts water, it is a pleasant gargle and mouth rinse. It is an effective agent for clearing candida overgrowth from the mouth, throat, and stomach. Used at full strength, it is excellent for combating vaginal yeast infection.

Latero Flora

(Bacillus laterosporus—B.O.D. Strain)

In 1981, a Southern California agriculturist visiting a remote part of Iceland discovered a native who had grown the most enormous, vibrantly colored, rich tasting vegetables he had ever seen. Inquiry revealed that the soil was like no other the agriculturist knew of! Untouched by pesticides, oxides of sulphur, carbon monoxide and related gasses, airborne chemicals, and all the other common pollutants which have ravaged most of the "civilized" world's soil, this small area contained remarkably pristine, pure soil. And vegetables grown in this soil appeared to impart remarkable health benefits to those who ate them regularly.

Excited to learn more, the agriculturist returned to the U.S.A. with enough of this unique soil to study it in depth. After a series of tests, the true secret of the soil's powers of growth and regeneration was revealed: the discovery of a unique strain of bacteria, Bacillus laterosporus.

The presence of large quantities of this microorganism in the soil apparently enhanced and bolstered plant growth. It was also theorized that individuals who ate these vegetables were not only receiving beneficial nutrients, but probably were consuming significant quantities of B. laterosporus itself.

Boyd O'Donnell, now president of Bio-Genesis Corp., was intrigued by the amazing properties of B. laterosporus and continued with several years of studies and development of the special strain. He then patented it as Bacillus laterosporus B.O.D., and named the product Latero Flora. The perfected methods for growth, stabilization, and preservation of the organism have been tested through human studies in which thousands of individuals have taken the product with beneficial results.

Latero Flora is extremely effective for individuals with gastro-intestinal disturbances, food allergies, and candidiasis hypersensitivity syndrome. Latero Flora normalizes the flora in the human digestive tract, aids in digestion and toxin elimination, and discourages the growth of yeast, fungi, and other pathogenic microorganisms.

As health professionals began to use Latero Flora, thousands of patients described dramatic feelings of improvement (confirmed by lab tests), and health organizations such as the Candida Research and Information Foundation gave glowing reports from trials. No other product in existence is as effective as Latero Flora in restoring the original, desirable, bacterial balance to human intestines, thus aiding in resolving many immuno-suppressed conditions.

Since early 1989 when Latero Flora was introduced commercially, continuously growing numbers of individuals, doctors, clinics and health care professionals have praised this product.

In separate testing, Dr. Luc DeSchepper, M.D., Ph.D., C.A., studied the "before and after" symptoms of 1,500 patients. These patients suffered from chronic fatigue, along with a wide variety of immunosuppressive symptoms. Dr. DeSchepper made his report in the Townsend Letter for Doctors:

> *Latero Flora has shown significant effectiveness in improving and in many cases eliminating gastrointestinal symptoms and food sensitivities, while enhancing the patient's digestive capacities . . . I am convinced that Latero Flora will play a very important role in fighting the scourge of this century—the suppression of our immune system.*

Travacid X (HCl)

Reprinted by permission from The Spotlight, *March 23, 1987*
by Tom Valentine

About 50 years ago, two physicians, supported by an abundance of original research, tried to tell the medical community that hydrochloric acid (HCl), the main constituent of stomach acid, held many keys to better health.

Both Dr. Burr Ferguson and William Bryant Guy were ignored by a medical Establishment dominated by a pharmaceutical industry bent on monopolizing all medical practice and its attendant promotion of "curative" substances.

Dr. Guy wrote exhaustively of using HCl as a therapy for many deadly diseases, especially about his clinical use of injections of dilute HCl into patients' veins.

Dr. Ferguson, credited with being the first M.D. to inject dilute HCl into the veins, showed that medical science went awry when it accepted the notions of Ehrlich (antibodies and side chains). Medical science erred again when it rejected much of the work of Elie Metchnikoff, who first propounded the theory of phagocytosis to explain natural immunity.

Metchnikoff named the white blood cells "phagocytes" because they are devourers of harmful, single-celled microbes.

June Perbohner, a devoted individual researcher, has studied the literature on HCl for more than a decade and provided the *Spotlight* this detailed exclusive.

"In 1936, Dr. Ferguson wrote 'Facts and Phagocytes,' in which he outlined the work of Metchnikoff and how it affected his researches into the HCl therapy," Perbohner said. "Metchnikoff earned half the Nobel Prize for [physiology and] medicine in 1908 for his work on phagocytes as presented in his book *Immunity in Infective Diseases.* Metchnikoff also advocated [the view] that most human ailments, and even 'old age' [senescence] were due to toxicities from intestinal putrefaction."

However, Metchnikoff and his followers, who included Louis Pasteur, could not explain why the phagocytes of one sick person function so well, while another person with the same disease succumbs.

"According to Dr. Ferguson," Perbohner noted, "bacteriolysis depends upon the acid balance of the cell, the electrical potential and [other factors]. Metchnikoff said that the white cells are acid in reaction, but he had never been able to identify what acid was responsible."

However, the medical Establishment had already latched onto the theory put forth by Ehrlich and "some 200 vaccines were made by laboratories of colleges and chemical houses in the application of this hypothetical system."

Ehrlich had astounding results in the treatment of syphilis, temporarily. His arsenic compounds worked until the germs became accustomed to the poison and mercury had to be added, then bismuth. The early signs that germs would adapt and build immunity to poisons didn't deter the drug industry from making more and more poisons.

A Better Stimulant

Figuring that Ehrlich had simply stimulated the phagocytes of Metchnikoff with his compounds, Ferguson sought a better chemical stimulant for the disease killing cells. He found it in nature's digestive acid.

The work of Ferguson and Guy established conclusively that simple hydrochloric acid, HCl, served to control the vital pH factors of the body systems. Ferguson also discovered that dilute HCl injected into the blood caused an increase in the oxygen supply of the blood.

However, medical science had moved away from Metchnikoff. Administering HCl intravenously required consummate skill, so Ferguson's HCl therapy vanished.

Perbohner has been instrumental in the creation of time-release HCl "caplets," which may be taken orally and may accomplish many of the purposes of the injectable HCl. Health food stores have long offered digestive HCl pills, even though the mainstream market prefers to sell antacids to curb stomach acid, which is erroneously believed to be part of the cause of ulcers.

Infectious diseases can get their start whenever there is a shortage of HCl in the system. Germs can survive heat and cold, but seldom can they survive strong acid. Ferguson provided 25 years of clinical researches to prove his HCl thesis.

Microbial infections, such as salmonellosis (food poisoning), are common and even epidemic among Americans today because of the diminished content of HCl in the gastric juices. A recent story in *Discover* magazine related how severe the problem of salmonella poisoning has become in the United States. Resistant strains of salmonella are proliferating in poultry and meats prepared in private homes, even more so than in public eateries.

The need for a strong stomach acid is quite apparent.

Healthy Lymph

Guy stressed the importance of the lymphatic system and how HCl was nature's way of keeping the lymph stream healthy and balanced. He presented his views on "the blockage of lymph channels due to changes in the hydrogenion content," and after five years of research showed that "most disease conditions, acute infections, anemias, metabolic disturbances, [etc.], are the direct result" of the changes in the pH of the lymphatic fluid (pH is a measure of acidity).

Guy pointed out how lymph "stasis" or blockage could seriously reduce the supply of oxygen to cells. He discovered that a subtle, but dangerous, form of lymph blockage occurred because of "mineral imbalance [and] pathological salts as seen in arthritis and gout."

Concern for the balance of minerals in the system has long been a hallmark of the so-called health faddists, while establishment medicine has downplayed the importance of such subtle balances of nature until recently.

"If oxygenation is reduced," Guy wrote, "the normal life in that group of cells slows down or ceases and abnormal metabolism begins."

Like many other great physicians of the 1920s and '30s, Guy knew that lack of oxygen for cell oxidation was the major cause of disease and aging.

Perbohner pointed out that "traveler's diarrhea" is one of the major health problems of the world and that it continues to pose puzzling problems for medical science.

"Numerous well-established facts on the relationship of reduced gastric acidity to intestinal bacterial and parasitic infection have been published," she told the *Spotlight*, "but evidence of the overall practical importance of gastric acid as it relates to immunity and intestinal bacterial and parasitic infections [is] incomplete."

She cited Dr. G. C. Cook, of the Department of Clinical and Tropical Medicine at the London School of Hygiene and Tropical Medicine, who commented as recently as 1985:

"It seems clear that far more attention was paid to gastric acid in the context of important defense mechanisms some three or four decades ago than is the case today. Altered emphasis has resulted from the explosion of interest in the immunological defense mechanisms which protect the gastrointestinal tract."

Cook also wrote: "Although the study of host defenses against intestinal infections is now dominated by immunologists, there is an important place for further research on gastric acidity in the context of infection."

Perbohner added: "It is timely to suggest that clinical research be undertaken on hydrogen and chloride ions in the context of so-called traveler's diarrhea and other related conditions."

Testimonials already abound to the efficacy of time-released HCl and sodium-chloride-oxygen compounds in the prevention of food poisoning and traveler's diarrhea. Both are ideas from the 1930s coming back.

It is interesting that a call can be made these days for more research into gastric acid. Why was so much quality research ignored 50 years ago?

Coenzyme Q10

Coenzyme Q10 (CoQ for short) is an important vitamin-like nutrient that functions biochemically as an anti-oxidant and free radical scavenger. But CoQ has a specific biochemical role of major importance. CoQ is essential for the production of cellular energy, and its role in producing energy in heart cells is of special interest. The steady stream of energy that is required to sustain life absolutely depends on each cell having adequate levels of CoQ.

This nutrient has become the focus of intense worldwide study. Hundreds of papers extolling the benefits of CoQ have been published in Japan, Europe, the former Soviet Union, and more recently in the U.S. CoQ is available from foods such as beef, spinach, and sardines. However, the body's ability to synthesize CoQ from foods diminishes with age and, furthermore, foods lose CoQ with processing and storage. CoQ is used throughout the world as a supplement to treat or prevent heart disease and high blood pressure, enhance the immune system, and slow the aging process. In Japan alone, more than 12 million people take daily doses of CoQ prescribed by their physicians for prevention and treatment of heart and circulatory disorders.

Animal studies conducted by Dr. Emile Bliznakov, Scientific Director of the Lupus Research Institute, have shown that mean life span can be increased significantly with CoQ. His experiments were conducted with mice whose ages were comparable to humans in their late sixties or early seventies. Within three to four months, the CoQ-supplemented mice were noticeable for their greater vigor and mobility, more lustrous hair, brighter eyes, and the absence of the normal signs of advanced age which were readily apparent in the control group. The life span of the CoQ-supplemented mice was twice as long as their predicted life expectancy.

The dual role of CoQ as an energy carrier and antioxidant may help account for its potential benefit for virtually every category of cell, tissue, and organ function. CoQ is a safe nutrient that is without significant side effects. CoQ has passed the toxicity studies required by the FDA for clinical trials in the United States. Topics of current research interest in CoQ include lupus, AIDS, diabetes, periodontal disease, *Candida albicans* infection, Parkinson's disease, and muscular dystrophy.

Benefits

- Coenzyme Q10 has proven of benefit in a variety of cardiovascular disorders.
- Enhances survival of heart tissue under low oxygen conditions and excessive loads.
- Has been shown in studies to have a stabilizing effect on heart rhythms.
- Can be effective in normalizing blood pressure in hypertensive individuals.
- May significantly enhance athletic performance.
- Helps improve oxygen transport and consumption and increase workload capacity.
- Has been shown to increase resistance to viral infections.
- Helps protect against chemically caused cancers.
- May dramatically increase antibody levels and stimulate the immune system.
- Has been proven effective in the treatment of obesity.
- Offers protection against inflammatory gum diseases.
- Has proven useful against diabetes and certain hearing disorders.
- Has been found effective in double-blind clinical studies in the treatment of AIDS.

Immuno-Quest

It has long been recognized that the healthy body's defense-mechanisms consist of white blood cells, lymph cells, and antibodies. White blood cells are found throughout the blood, serving to destroy bacteria, while lymph cells destroy viruses and antibodies, protecting us from foreign proteins and matter that are associated with bacteria.

Viruses and bacteria are opportunistic living organisms that prey upon us when our immune system is weak. Factors that can affect our immunity are poor diet, stress, lack of exercise, tobacco and alcohol use, and even some medications. The temperature, pH, and low energy level of our body when we are in a run-down state creates the perfect environment for viruses and bacteria to flourish. When they proliferate sufficiently, our body's immune defenses break down and we develop the physical symptoms of illness. Such illnesses include the common cold and flu, and the range of infections from herpes to AIDS.

Drugs relieve only the physical symptoms of infection, oftentimes making the situation worse by killing the bacteria and leaving their dead bodies in our tissues to serve as breeding material for new bacteria and viruses. This creates a vicious cycle of illness until our immune defense system becomes damaged and chronic disease sets in. Such diseases include allergies, lupus, arthritis, chronic infections, and cancer.

Scientists are daily gaining a better understanding of the immune system and what it takes to biochemically aid and support its function. Many of these biochemical components are being found in vitamins, minerals and herbs, nutrients that are essential in nourishing our bodies.

Immuno-Quest combines essential nutrients to reinforce and stimulate our bodily defenses. These are as follows:

Vitamin C: This essential vitamin is always depleted in the tissues during illness. It stimulates the production of antibodies and white blood cells, and is deadly to all viruses.

It is also important to the body's recuperative powers and vascular strength.

Vitamin A: Vitamin A is also essential to the production of antibodies, white blood cells and lymphocytes. As with Vitamin C, the level of Vitamin A drops sharply during infections. Vitamin A also promotes the repair of tissues damaged by illness and stress.

Zinc: Experiments performed by DuPont scientists showed that by adding zinc to tissue cultures the formation of bacteria and viruses was immediately inhibited. Zinc has been widely used commercially in antibacterial preparations because of its bacterial inhibiting properties. Zinc is one of our most important minerals, having over 32 functions in our bodies.

Pantothenic Acid (Vitamin B5): This nutrient is necessary for the production of cortisone, an anti-inflammatory agent in the body. Vitamins B5 and B6 also help to promote production of antibodies and white blood cells.

Vitamin B12 and *RNA*: These two nutrients support the body as antitoxins during chronic infections such as mononucleosis and hepatitis. Their effect is enhanced by Vitamins C and A, bioflavonoids, and other nutrients.

Coenzyme Q10: This nutrient is found in all tissues and has many functions, primarily antioxidant in nature. Studies have shown that it retards cellular destruction from aging and stress, thus enhancing healing. Other studies have shown that supplemental Coenzyme Q10 increases immunoglobulin and the germ-killing ability of white blood cells.

L-Lysine: An essential amino acid, L-lysine is principally an antiviral agent. It has been used successfully in the treatment of herpes and herpeto-viruses such as chicken pox. Combined with Coenzyme Q10 and Vitamin C, L-lysine has a synergistic effect.

Glandular Extracts: Commonly known as protomorphigens, freeze-dried glandulars have been widely used. In medicine, thyroid extract is used quite frequently. In nutrition, glandulars add micronutrients that support the activity of their targeted gland. The immune glands are the thymus, spleen, lymph, and lung.

Herbal Concentrates: Echinacea is one of the most outstanding herbs for the immune system, activating white blood and lymph cells. It is an effective antibacterial and antiviral agent possessing similar activity to interferon. It is also a good blood purifier, toning those organs that filter impurities from the blood. Alfalfa, chlorophyll, and kelp are powerful herbs that act to normalize the pH balance, creating a nutritional environment for proper vitamin and mineral absorption. These herbs also help to "sweeten" the digestive tract, removing and neutralizing toxic mucous.

Natur-Earth

An Amazing New Breakthrough in Immune Stimulation and Healing

Scientists are working on "grooming" various non-native microorganisms to perform specific tasks in the human body, such as destroying certain viruses, or stimulating specific functions within the immune system. In several instances, great strides have been made in these areas—one of which has been in the development and use of *soil-based microorganisms* for promoting overall healing in human beings, as well as for stimulating powerful responses unlike anything ever reported.

Later you will learn the inside details on a unique new immune-therapeutic product called Natur-Earth, which utilizes soil-based microorganisms in its makeup. But first, here's a brief explanation of what soil-based microorganisms are, and what they do.

SBOs in the Human Diet

Most Americans don't realize it, but many forms of SBOs, as well as their enzyme, hormone, and nutrient byproducts, are unknowingly ingested into the human system—with very beneficial effects—when fresh raw fruits and vegetables are eaten. This was especially true in the nineteenth century, when America was basically one large rural farming community and the ingestion of fresh raw fruits and vegetables—often straight from the fields or directly from family gardens—was commonplace.

Today, however, human ingestion of SBOs and their beneficial byproducts is far less common. This is because modern agricultural techniques (including the over-application of powerful pesticides, fungicides, and germicidal agents) and heat-based food processing techniques tend to kill off SBOs on fruits and vegetables, as well as destroy the beneficial enzyme, hormone, and nutrient by-products normally released by SBOs

139

and absorbed by the food plants as part of the normal growth cycle. Nonetheless, SBOs and their beneficial by-products still manage to find their way into the human system today in this country, though with far less frequency than in times past.

It is because of this that a number of nutritionists working on the cutting edge of orthomolecular medicine now speculate that the declining digestive intake of SBOs and their enzyme, hormone, and nutrient by-products is one of the chief reasons Americans tend to experience far more bowel and digestive systems problems than do the people of other countries, where modern high-tech farming and food processing techniques have yet to replace family farms and gardens. In other countries, SBO intake is markedly higher via the intake of fresh raw plant life, and digestive tract problems are correspondingly lower!

The Making of Natur-Earth

In the late 1980s a reclusive scientist by the name of Peter Smith was on a trip overseas. While hiking through a pristine area of a foreign country [which, to this day, he won't name— Ed.], he spotted some large clumps on the ground, which he recognized as huge colonies of soil-based microorganisms. Smith was intrigued by the unusual nature of what he saw, and brought some of the microorganisms back into the United States for research and experimentation. Later, he returned several times to the original location to obtain additional samples.

For the next few years, Smith conducted phased studies of the soil-based microorganisms he had discovered. Phase #1 was to identify the various strains of SBOs found living in the clumps. Phase #2 was to determine if the SBOs were toxic or pathogenic. Phase #3 was to ascertain what, if any, beneficial value these soil-based bacteria might be able to impart to living things, particularly animals and humans.

After considerable painstaking and detailed research, the specific strains of soil-based bacilli Smith had discovered were identified. Toxicity tests proved negative on fingerling fish. In fact, far from being harmed, the fish began rapidly increasing in size when taking the bacteria. Toxicity tests were then carefully conducted on rodents and other members of the animal kingdom with equally positive results. There was nothing in the bacteria toxic to animals. At the same time, extensive botany tests were conducted which showed that the bacteria were amazingly beneficial to plants and soil.

Smith became the first human being to use the bacterial culture himself—first using it topically on open wounds, and later ingesting it. Again there were no toxic reactions to the bacteria, and there were no harmful side effects. In fact, it seemed to give increasingly positive health results as more and more of the organisms were consumed.

According to the source material we were able to obtain for this report, Smith's research was conducted in the laboratories of several major California universities. He collaborated with top professors and other research experts, and was able to utilize the facilities of the laboratories freely, as well as the computer data banks.

In the course of his research and experimentation, Smith and his laboratory coworkers were able to perfect a process for selectively breeding superior strains of the tiny microorganism, as well as for "grooming" them until they had a culture that, when ingested by humans, produced very specific and quite startling healing and immune-stimulating results, with absolutely no toxic effects or other unwanted side effects. The combined corporate effort of Smith and his university colleagues ultimately resulted in the development of the amazing Natur-Earth food supplement product.

Natur-Earth is manufactured as a gray-black powder. The powder, which is composed chiefly of a broad array of specific micronutrients and phytoplankton, acts as a *substrate* for live soil-based microorganisms. Through a special process, the SBOs are kept in a dormant state within the powder, and do not become active until introduced into a aqueous solution such as water or juice. Because of this, Natur-Earth boasts a shelf-life of over five years at room temperature, and even longer if refrigerated.

Secret Process

In the course of our research on this product, we discovered that Smith holds no patent to Natur-Earth, nor to the various processes he developed in order to selectively breed and "groom" the soil-based microorganisms. Nor has he patented his technique for putting the organisms into the dormant state which gives them such an unusually long shelf life. According to our sources, this is because he wants to prevent his product from being duplicated or stolen.

To this day, Smith will not identify the original soil-based organisms he discovered, nor discuss his processes for selectively breeding and grooming the superior strains from the original cultures.

Dramatic Healing Results!

Nonetheless, in spite of all the secrecy surrounding Natur-Earth, the product has enjoyed over 12 years of continuous—albeit very quiet—use by the relatively small number of people who have been fortunate enough to hear about it. In that time, no toxic side effects have ever been reported. What *has* been reported over the course of the past 12 years are dramatic cases of remission from some of the most serious illnesses and chronic degenerative diseases known to man, including candida.

What's more, users of Natur-Earth report numerous other ongoing health benefits, such as virtual immunity from colds and flu, stronger digestive capabilities, elimination of constipation and other chronic digestive disorders, increased and/or stabilized metabolism, increased energy levels, increased physical strength, greater resistance to inflammation, quicker resistance to infection, quicker healing of wounds, increased mental clarity, and much, much more.

We were able to examine the results of specific tests, as well as scientific laboratory analysis performed on the product, which revealed the specific actions through which Natur-Earth is able to stabilize the metabolism in human beings, radically boost nutritional assimilation, and simultaneously amplify the human immune system to such a degree that illness and disease can be warded off indefinitely, and even reversed if already in progress.

This information gives a startling insight into what makes Natur-Earth such a remarkable therapeutic product. We'll give you some of the specific details in just a moment, but first, here's a basic outline of how Natur-Earth works when taken orally, as well as a brief description of the five main functions of the SBOs contained in Natur-Earth.

How It Works: A Basic Outline

When Natur-Earth is ingested, it moves from the stomach to the intestinal tract and forms colonies of beneficial SBOs along the way, which attach themselves to the intestinal wall. Then, as food works its way through the gastrointestinal system, it drags some of the bacteria from these colonies further "down the line," these bacteria also attaching to the intestinal wall. Within a short period of time, the microorganism attachment to the intestinal wall encompasses literally the entire length of the gastrointestinal tract.

The SBOs in Natur-Earth grow and multiply into large colonies wherever they attach to the intestinal wall. Once established, they quickly begin producing an environment which dramatically stimulates the body's ability to absorb and utilize crucial nutrients, while simultaneously ridding the intestinal tract of both putrefaction and pathogenic (i.e., disease-causing) organisms. Here are five of the main functions conducted by the SBOs once they are integrated into the human intestinal system through ingestion as a food supplement.

Function #1: Once the SBOs have established their colonies in the digestive tract, they immediately begin eliminating all accumulated putrefaction in which harmful pathogenic organisms thrive. The SBOs have the ability to get in behind putrefaction that has stuck to the walls of the colon and other areas of the intestinal tract and devour it. Excess putrefaction is dislodged by the SBOs and then flushed out of the intestinal tract by the normal eliminative process.

Function #2: The SBOs also go to work breaking down hydrocarbons. With this unique ability, all foods are broken down into their most basic elements, allowing almost total absorption through the digestive system, thereby dramatically increasing overall nutrition and rapidly enhancing cellular growth and development. This process also vastly aids the digestive system in the process of elimination because of the unusually thorough and complete manner in which foods are broken down by the SBOs. As a major side benefit, constipation is eliminated almost overnight.

Function #3: While in the digestive tract, the SBOs produce specific proteins which act as antigens. These in turn stimulate the immune system to produce huge quantities of antibodies over and above that which the immune system would normally have available for use. This vastly increased antibody output dramatically amplifies the immune system's ability to ward off disease and illness. Plus, it enhances the immune system's ability to battle virtually any disease or illness already afflicting the body. Because of this factor, which we'll explain in depth, many individuals using Natur-Earth have reported amazing healing results from diseases.

Function #4: The SBOs are extremely aggressive against pathological molds, yeast, fungi, and viruses. They quickly engulf and ingest harmful microbes such as *Candida Albicans*, *Candida Parasylois*, *Penicillin Frequency*, *Penicillin Natatum*,

Muco Rasmosue, Aspergillus Niger, and many others, which would otherwise infect the body and cause serious illness and even chronic degenerative disease. In eliminating pathogenic microbes, the SBOs end up allowing the overworked immune system to rest and gain strength.

Function #5: The SBOs work in a symbiotic relation to somatic cells. They metabolize proteins for the cells and simultaneously help rid them of toxic wastes, thereby dramatically boosting normal cellular functions which are the very basis of all human health.

Chiefly because of these five specific functions of the SBOs contained in Natur-Earth, dramatic healing and immune-stimulation are being achieved for people around the world who are quietly using this unique and exclusive new therapeutic food supplement. But the truly fascinating immune-stimulating effects of the SBOs can only be fully realized when one looks at the data produced by ongoing laboratory tests being conducted by some of the world's top scientists and immune system experts.

Natur-Earth and the Human Immune System: The Inside Details

When I first heard about this product, well frankly, I thought to myself 'this is probably just snake oil.' I was very suspicious. Then I heard how people with arthritis were being helped, and people with Lou Gehrig's disease. And people with various kinds of cancer. So I went out to Los Angeles and interviewed people who had used it, and looked at their medical histories, and I became a believer . . . Without a doubt, people are being helped.
                                        —Dr. Don Boys, Ph.D.

I didn't believe what I was reading about this product. I started studying it. Soon, I could see the logic behind how and why it works. The first patient we put on this product was a man with a serious bladder and kidney infection, who also had enlargement of the prostate and was scheduled for prostate surgery. Within four days of taking the product there was no more infection, so the surgery was temporarily postponed. Two weeks later the patient was re-examined and there was no more enlargement of the prostrate. The surgery was cancelled . . . This is just one example of the amazing results we've witnessed with this product. We've recorded remissions from various diseases beginning within three days to four weeks after using this product . . . Cancers, Parkinson's disease, glaucoma, nervous disorders, high cholesterol levels, and many other conditions and diseases have responded successfully to this product.

—Dr. Phyllis Wilson Confer
Marko, Indiana

I had breast cancer that had metastasized to the bone. By the time it was found, it was simply too late for conventional therapy. It was advanced to the point of being a death sentence. I was in a lot of pain . . . I started taking the product in November, and within weeks I felt decreased pain—in fact, about 95 percent less pain. Since then the central mass of cancer in my breast has decreased from a two-and-one-half-inch mass to the size of a small pea.

—Dr. A. Johnson (City/State withheld on request)

I have been afflicted with arthritis for nearly 20 years, and in recent years have had to use a wheelchair to get around the house. I started taking this product twice daily in orange juice. It took about two or three weeks for the pain to go away. I find it better to take than the pills and other medication the doctors give me, as there are no *side effects. The doctor's medicine gave me an ulcer. But this product is the best thing I've ever tried.*

—I. C. (age 74), Texas

My health for over one month's time was very poor. I was operating on about 25 to 50 percent of my energy level. I had swollen glands and a sore throat . . . The doctor's statement—'you just have to ride it out because I have nothing to give you to make you feel better.' I spoke with my neighbor, and he told me about your product. He gave me some to try, told me to take it twice a day. Within 12 hours my sore throat was gone, and 24 hours later my glands stopped hurting, and within 48 hours my energy level was back to normal! It was definitely a miracle cure for me.

—M. M., California

For 13 years I wrestled to find a way to stabilize and hopefully heal one of my children who had uncontrollable epilepsy which traditional Western medication did not help. Last year, while visiting with a man who has been called one of the top five biochemists in the world, at his prestigious clinic in Key Biscayne, Florida, I was introduced to a product he dubbed 'black gold' . . . When I began giving my epileptic child this product, the petit mal seizures, which had been continuous for 13 years, stopped literally overnight . . . Could these beneficial microorganisms emit substances which are useful to the human intestine, and work against foreign matter or other debris found in the intestine? Could these microorganisms, as they grow in colonies, emit substances which stimulate the body's response to produce antibodies which are an immune simulator, which in turn amplify and stabilize the body's immune system? All I know for

sure is that this product knocked out my child's petit mal seizures, and has increased my energy level and stamina.
—R. E. McMaster
Publisher, *The Reaper*

As we've stated earlier, the amazing immune-stimulating benefits produced by the actions of the SBOs in Natur-Earth have been demonstrated in literally hundreds of individual cases over the past 12 years. The examples above are just a small fraction of personal testimonials from users of this amazing product. Clinical trials now underway in Mexico, Venezuela, Spain, and other countries will provide even more detailed documentation of the amazing healing effects being experienced by individuals when this product is used regularly.

In the meantime, laboratory examinations have provided some fascinating in-depth insights into how it works in the human body, and why such dramatic healing and immune-stimulation benefits are being experienced by so many individuals with such a diversity of illnesses and disease.

In the course of laboratory analysis, three totally unique immune-stimulation actions have been discovered. Each of these three specific actions constitute major new breakthroughs in orthomolecular medicine that offer profound ramifications for modern medical science. To our knowledge, medical science so far has produced nothing that can duplicate these three extremely powerful immune-stimulating actions, which are as follows:

Action #1: Stimulation of the Body's Natural Alpha Interferon Production
According to Dr. Peter Rothschild, who has conducted in-depth laboratory analysis of Natur-Earth and the beneficial SBOs, once they are firmly established in the gastrointestinal tract, they stimulate the body's own natural production of *alpha-interferon.*

Alpha-interferon is a paramount polypeptide—a protein form molecule—that was discovered in the human body in 1956 and has been proven to be a key regulator of the human immune response. Since its discovery, it has been universally acknowledged by science that the development of a widely useable man-made form of alpha-interferon would embody profound hope for the cure of many diseases in the future. Unfortunately, to date science has failed to develop a form of alpha-interferon that could live up to the high expectations held for it since its discovery in the human body.

Medical science's recombinantly-derived alpha-interferon has limited applications, with limited beneficial effects. For one, the extreme dosages (i.e., multi-million unit daily doses) required in order to stimulate immune response in humans have proven to be highly toxic. Achieving a pure form of the element has also been a major problem for medical science. What's more, the man-made alpha-interferon has proven to be prohibitively costly to manufacture and utilize, with individual treatments costing thousands upon thousands of dollars.

Additionally distressing is the fact that the recombinantly-derived interferons used by medical science today have only a single species of alpha-interferon which exerts a very low immune-stimulation response, whereas the interferons produced naturally by the human body are *multi-species* in nature. The healthy human leukocyte cell can produce up to *twenty* different sub-species of alpha-interferon and exert an *extremely aggressive* immune response.

Moreover, science now knows that the reason the human body produces so many different subspecies of alpha-interferon is because different subspecies are required to protect cells against different viruses and other antigens. No single subspecies of endogenous (i.e., body-produced) alpha-interferon can protect the human system against the variety of harmful invaders with which it must regularly contend. Therefore, the limited immune benefits of the expensive, single-species alpha-interferon produced by medical science simply cannot hold a candle to the vast immune benefits of the multi-species of alpha-interferon produced naturally by the human body itself.

In laboratory tests performed by Dr. Rothschild, the actions of the soil-based organisms contained in Natur-Earth have been shown to uniquely stimulate the human body's own production *of not less than 16 of the possible 20 subspecies of natural human alpha-interferon!* Dr. Rothschild speculates that it is this incredible stimulation of the body's production of its own natural alpha-interferon which has caused Natur-Earth to be so highly effective in the treatment of a wide variety of chronic degenerative diseases such as chronic fatigue syndrome, viral herpes, hepatitis-B and C, influenza, and much more. To date, we know of no other product which can achieve such a profound immune-stimulating action.

What's more, according to Dr. Rothschild, "The anti-viral activity stimulated by the SBOs in Natur-Earth is even more clear, for the virus-antagonistic effect of alpha-interferon has long been documented by worldwide scientific investigation . . . *Our research has identified over 50 different immune modulating effects to date* . . . This research has produced ample evidence indicating Natur-Earth exerts a potent immune-modulatory influence with significant clinical benefits to patients who suffer from a variety of viral aggressions or other immunopathic, degenerative conditions."

Additionally, Dr. Rothschild found that, "Since Natur-Earth does not contain any toxic, addictive or otherwise dangerous substance, it is totally harmless and provides the particular elements required for stimulating both the body's T-cell production and their quality. It also eliminates the need for poisonously high-dose and inordinately expensive alpha-interferon injections."

In short, it now appears that the SBOs in Natur-Earth are unique in that their actions in the human gastrointestinal tract are somehow *able to stimulate the body's own production of the vast majority of subspecies of its own natural alpha-interferon,* thereby dramatically enhancing the immune system's ability to ward off illness and disease. T-lymphocyte production is greatly boosted and the anti-viral activity of the immune system is vastly stimulated as a direct effect of increased alpha-interferon production.

What's more, because the alpha-interferon produced as a result of the ingestion of Natur-Earth is endogenous, it is also far more assimilable by the human immune system than medical science's recombinantly-derived alpha-interferon. And the overwhelming problems of purity and toxicity are completely eliminated through the use of Natur-Earth, since it merely stimulates the body to produce its own naturally pure forms.

Lastly, instead of medical science having to indulge in vastly ineffective immune system treatments costing thousands upon thousands of dollars as they do now with their recombinantly-derived alpha-interferon, dramatic and highly effective immune-stimulating results can be achieved in the human body for a tiny fraction of the cost through the use of Natur-Earth!

Action #2: Stimulation of B-lymphocytes and Related Antibody Production

Once established in the gastrointestinal tract, the SBOs in Natur-Earth quickly begin producing a protein biomass which the body reacts to as an antigen (i.e., a foreign substance). In response to the antigenic biomass, the body immediately begins producing large quantities of *B-lymphocytes*, which in turn produce large quantities of *antibodies*.

According to Dr. Rothschild's extensive laboratory experimentation and analysis, the antibodies produced by the immune system in reaction to the antigenic biomass from the SBOs are *extremely unique* in that they are "non-addressed" antibodies. That is, they have not been "pre-programmed" by the immune system to attack any specific infection or pathogenic agent.

Instead, huge pools of antibodies are produced as long as the SBOs are ingested on a regular basis, *and they are kept in reserve by the body for use whenever needed by the immune system*. If an actual infection takes hold, or a specific pathogen invades the body, the immune system then instantly—at a moment's notice—"imprints" this large reservoir of otherwise innocuous antibodies with the precise information needed to attack the specific infection or pathogenic agent at hand. Then, quite rapidly and with incredible effectiveness, the antibodies go to work attacking the infection or pathogen at once, and wipe it out.

As explained by Dr. Rothschild, "The beauty of it all is that this huge reservoir of extra antibodies is always on hand for the immune system to utilize; as long as the individual is ingesting the SBOs regularly, the effectiveness of the human immune system is vastly enhanced. This extra contingent of antibodies is always there to attack infection, therefore the immune system does not have to work anywhere near as hard as it normally would to fight off infection."

In a nutshell, it appears that the SBOs in Natur-Earth stimulate the human immune system to produce huge pools of extra antibodies—unique, *nonspecific* antibodies which the immune system can encode whenever necessary to fight off many different types of infection or pathogenic agents. Thanks to these billions of extra antibodies, the human system can be kept far safer from infection or invading pathogens than ever before. With this unusual immuno-stimulatory effect, the human body can now act far more effectively to protect itself from infection or invading pathogens.

Action #3: Crucial Lactoferrin Supplementation
to the Human Body
Dr. Rothschild has discovered that one of the most amazing aspects of the SBOs used in Natur-Earth is their ability to produce lactoferrin in the human body as a by-product of their

metabolism. Lactoferrin, an iron-binding protein, is specifically utilized to retrieve iron from the foods we ingest, and then deliver the iron wherever it is needed by the body. Because the affinity of lactoferrin for iron is very high, it is able to retain and transport iron even through the harsh gastric environment, so it can be delivered to the small intestine where it is absorbed by specific receptors on the epithelial cells.

Unfortunately, lactoferrin levels are often not high enough in the human body for a variety of reasons. As a consequence, many people have trouble properly assimilating the iron they've ingested through the foods they eat. And because the body is not assimilating iron properly, symptoms of *iron deficiency* appear, even though plenty of iron is being ingested on a daily basis.

This problem is further compounded today because Americans are literally inundated with advertisements from vitamin manufacturers telling them they need to take iron supplements. What's more, many doctors tell their patients they are suffering from "iron poor blood" and need to ingest supplemental iron tablets. In reality, what most Americans need to do is increase their bodily levels of lactoferrin, so that the iron from the foods they eat—*which is more than adequate for the human system*—is more thoroughly assimilated.

In fact, as Dr. Peter Rothschild points out in his recently published research report on the *Biology of Lactoferrin*, "Of the 750 million people who suffer from iron deficiency symptoms, less than half of them suffer from any actual lack of iron in their diet." Instead, he explains, their iron deficiency symptoms are due chiefly to metabolic problems (such as those caused by insufficient levels of lactoferrin) that hinder the assimilation of iron from the food they eat, or because of the low bio-accessibility of the ingested iron.

Of course, this creates a serious problem when individuals suffering from alleged "iron deficiency" begin taking iron supplements. The additional iron being ingested does absolutely nothing to alleviate the iron deficiency symptoms because it, too, remains unassimilated by the body. As a result, the body becomes inundated with iron that it simply cannot assimilate and utilize.

Worse yet, excess iron soon begins to support the growth of infectious agents throughout the human body, due to the fact that harmful bacteria, yeasts, viruses, and other parasites have a continuous metabolic need for iron, and tend to thrive in an iron-rich environment!

On the other hand, when iron is carried through the body by lactoferrin, as it is meant to be, more than 95 percent of it is assimilable. Lactoferrin carries the iron directly to specific receptor sites in the body where it can be absorbed and utilized. Because it is attached to lactoferrin, iron cannot be absorbed and utilized by the bacteria, viruses, yeasts, and other harmful parasites that require it for their metabolism.

What all of this means, according to Dr. Rothschild, is that "One of lactoferrin's primary functions in the human body is to act as a first line of defense against all invading pathogens."

In short, lactoferrin not only makes the iron we absorb from food readily assimilable by the human body (thereby eliminating iron deficiency symptoms), it also deprives infectious organisms of this crucial element needed for their survival and growth. In a sense, it *starves to death* harmful organisms in the human body by depriving them of iron, thus short-circuiting their metabolic functions!

As mentioned earlier, Dr. Rothschild's research has shown that the SBOs in Natur-Earth produce lactoferrin in the human body as a result of their own metabolism. So by taking Natur-Earth regularly, your body will be far better able to absorb, assimilate, and utilize the iron supplied by the food you eat. Iron supplements should become completely unnecessary, once your body begins taking advantage of the increased levels of lactoferrin supplied by Natur-Earth, which reduces fatigue.

Summary of Natur-Earth's Unique Immune-Stimulating Actions

In summary, the beneficial SBOs used in Natur-Earth provide an exclusive triple action level of immune-stimulation that is not available through any other therapeutic development we know of.

1. They stimulate the body's own natural alpha-interferon production, thereby providing markedly increased T-lymphocyte levels, dramatically increased viral resistance, and a high level of protection against chronic degenerative disease unattainable by modern medical science up until now;

2. They also stimulate the production of crucial B-lymphocytes and related antibodies, providing the immune system with a huge extra reservoir of anti-pathogenic defense organisms that are available for use at a moment's notice; and,

3. They directly produce much needed lactoferrin for the human body, which helps protect it from invading pathogens by depriving them of the iron they need in order to survive in the human system.

More Amazing Therapeutic Benefits

In addition to all of these immuno-therapeutic benefits, the SBOs in Natur-Earth also produce and/or stimulate a vast number of other important health-related benefits. Dr. Rothschild's laboratory research on Natur-Earth has shown that it produces at least 50 distinct beneficial immune-modeling effects alone. In addition, it also directly produces and/or stimulates a number of crucial cellular health benefits.

Stimulates Cellular Self-Repair

For example, as a result of their action in the human system, the SBOs contained in Natur-Earth produce a wide array of DNA with their correspondent RNA. The DNA/RNA produced by the SBOs is of the specific type which is very desirable for the human body, because it carries naturally-coded instructions for the activation of self-repair in certain human cells.

It is believed that this specific factor is the reason many users of Natur-Earth have reported incredible accelerations of wound healing, particularly in regard to severe skin burns, ulcers, surgical incisions, and even wounds that had become infected. Apparently, the DNA/RNA produced by the SBOs helps aid the body in activating cellular self-repair by making available a pool of extra DNA/RNA that is immediately available to the cells, and can go right to work whenever injury occurs.

Provides Powerful Anti-Oxidants

But the therapeutic benefits don't end with the production of cell-repairing DNA and RNA. Another interesting action of the SBOs in Natur-Earth is that they produce SOD (Super Oxide Dismutase) as a by-product of their metabolism in the human system. SOD is a powerful enzyme and cellular anti-oxidant that acts as a super-scavenger of dangerous free radicals by ferreting out and destroying them throughout the body.

This is important, because free radicals are highly active and unstable and will attack any molecule in the body. Organ or tissue damage can occur whenever production of free radicals exceeds that of scavenger enzymes, such as SOD, which are the first-line defense system of the body's tissues.

But because very few foods contain SOD, our bodies are often deficient in this all-important enzyme. Thus, the damaging effects of free radicals (such as superoxide radical O2, which induce cancer and a variety of painful inflammatory diseases as well) often goes unchecked. By introducing SOD into the human system on a regular basis, such as through the use of Natur-Earth, many dangerous free radicals can be easily extinguished before they harm the cells.

What's more, studies conducted at Johns Hopkins University have shown that SOD eliminates or greatly reduces tissue damage in the heart (particularly after a heart attack). Plus, it can also reduce tissue damage in the kidneys, the intestines, the pancreas, and the skin. This is because the enzymatic activity of SOD greatly increases the efficiency of energy production within the cells of organ tissues, allowing them to nourish and repair themselves at a more efficient and effective rate.

By using Natur-Earth on a regular basis, your body will be assured of receiving beneficial amounts of this all-important enzyme, as well as literally dozens of others.

Corrects Nutrient Absorption Deficiencies

In addition to all of the startling health benefits detailed above, Natur-Earth also provides a unique level of micronutrient support of the human body unparalleled in any other therapeutic product we've ever investigated. More importantly, this special level of micronutrient support acts to correct nutrient absorption deficiencies in the body, *thereby giving the human system the ability to obtain all of the nutrients it needs from daily food intake*, rather than having to depend upon a plethora of nutrient supplements. Here's how it works.

Most nutrient supplement products are based upon the premise that the human body is simply not getting enough nutrients from the food it ingests on a daily basis. Therefore, most of today's nutrient supplement products are designed to inundate the body with medium-to-large dosages of nutrients in order to make up for the alleged deficit of nutrients in the food supply.

But this form of nutrient supplementation rarely works well because the premise it is based upon is patently false. As Dr. Rothschild points out in his recent research report entitled *Bioactive Micronutrient Minerals: Biological Response Modifiers*,

"A specific or multiple mineral deficit in a human body usually does NOT imply that there is a corresponding deficit of these minerals in the individual's daily nutrition . . . Instead, the real problem in such individuals is a chronic absorption deficiency."

In other words, as a general rule there are plenty of nutrients in the foods we eat, but due to aging, abuse or other factors, our bodies are having a difficult time *absorbing* these nutrients. So, in reality, flooding the human body with high-dose nutrient supplements is of little benefit because the whole problem in the first place is the body's inability to properly absorb nutrients!

That's where Natur-Earth is distinctly different—and far more effective—than all other nutrient supplements. Instead of inundating the body with overly-high levels of supplemental nutrients, it instead provides a wide array of key nutrients in special *micronutrient dosages*. These tiny microscopic dosages are so easy to assimilate that they act as veritable *blueprints* for the body, showing it how to properly absorb other nutrients already available in quite adequate levels through daily food intake.

In a very real sense, the special microscopic dosages of nutrients supplied in Natur-Earth act as biological "data," literally providing the cells of the human body with an "absorption pattern" which shows them how to effectively assimilate and utilize the higher levels of nutrients contained in most foods.

Dr. Rothschild's research has revealed that some of the key micronutrients made available to the body through the ingestion of Natur-Earth are actually produced as by-products of the metabolism of the SBOs once they enter the body. Other micronutrients are contained *within the SBOs themselves*, and are made available to the human body as the SBOs die off and the body digests them. And still other micronutrients are contained in the freshly-cultivated phyto-plankton (i.e., blue-green algae) cells used in Natur-Earth as a nutrient substrate.

PRODUCTS FOR CANDIDA CONTROL

There are at least 71 naturally occurring nutrients available in Natur-Earth, or provided as a by-product of the metabolism of the SBOs contained in the product. These include numerous beneficial pigments such as chlorophyll and phytocyanin, plus amino acids, vitamins (including the crucial B_{12}), minerals, key enzymes (including SOD and bromelain), nucleic acids, proteins, and more.

Additionally, Natur-Earth contains the immune-stimulating, cancer-preventing, vitamin A precursor known as beta-carotene. It also supplies the body with Gamma Linolenic Acid (GLA), which is one of the essential fatty acids without which the body could not produce hormones. In fact, without GLA the endocrine system cannot even function. [Note the human body is unable to synthesize GLA, and often has a hard time extracting it from foods. Natur-Earth solves this problem completely.]

These nutrients are available in such microscopic dosages that they are rapidly and easily absorbed into the human cellular system, and thereby act as *biological response modifiers*— i.e., they literally help the body modify its ability to absorb larger dosages of nutrients from natural food sources.

No other product we know of today can do this. The micronutrients supplied in Natur-Earth literally "guide" your system in the proper absorption of nutrients from foods, and thereby dramatically increase your body's ability to grow and heal itself. By taking Natur-Earth, along with maintaining a healthy daily diet, your body will have all the nutritional support necessary for cellular repair and growth, thereby enabling it to be more effective in warding off illness and disease.

The SBOs in Natur-Earth are not permanent residents of the intestines. They are there temporarily during therapy and will remain on an active basis for about forty-eight hours if the product is no longer taken. Best results are received when taken every day, as they will colonize on the intestinal wall, doubling themselves every twenty minutes. The SBOs grow very fast and will eat away the attachment sites of candida, hardened mucus, and wastes that are stuck to the intestinal wall, and within pockets or diverticuli found within the colon. Not only do SBOs destroy candida from the inside out, but cause large pieces of it to fall away from the wall of the intestine, thereby quickening its removal.

Observing the results of using Natur-Earth for twelve years, it was shown to be more effective in removing candida, molds, fungus, and negative microorganisms from the body than any other nutritional supplement. The ability for SBOs to grow at a rapid pace and literally devour and destroy a yeast infection throughout the entire body makes this product indispensable for the permanent removal of a candida condition. However, the complimentary ability to encourage immuno-responsive T-cells, anti-bodies, and alpha-interferon to massively accumulate within the systems of the body allows systemic candida that may be in the blood, organs, brain, and tissues to also be neutralized and removed. This again is a remarkable accomplishment when you consider there is little available in systemic remedies for candida.

The soil-based microorganisms in Natur-Earth are thoroughbreds. Peter Smith discovered the original organism, bred and groomed them, so to speak, and eliminated from them any undesirable elements. When you take a capsule of Natur-Earth, you are taking a thoroughbred selection—highly selected colonies of beneficial soil-based organisms. Peter Smith bred these organisms to perfection, where the production of undesirable elements is zero—absolutely zero! That's why I call him a genius.
—Dr. Peter Rothschild

A Major New Weapon against Viruses, Candida, Allergies

by Dr. Robert W. Bradford, President
Bradford Research Institute

Dioxychlor®, one of a class of inorganic oxidants, has been found useful against the three major classes of infective agents — virus, bacteria, and fungi—and to have tremendous potential use in such refractory conditions as acquired immune deficiency syndrome (AIDS). It is also extremely effective against an impressive array of viral, bacterial, and fungal infections, including demonstrated inhibition of *Candida albicans*.

University research has indicated the in vitro effectiveness of Dioxychlor—the premier inorganic oxidant—against the putative "AIDS virus" (HTLV-III/HIV), hepatitis-B, Epstein-Barr virus, cytomegalovirus, polio, and other viral strains. Ongoing in vivo research by the Mexican division of the Bradford Research Institute has confirmed substantial effectiveness against candida, Epstein-Barr, and conditions related to AIDS and AIDS-Related Complex (ARC), Universal Reactor Syndrome (URS), and many lesser conditions.

At the same time, the use of Dioxychlor and the development of specialized microscopy have helped establish what we may call "the pleomorphic foundation of environmental illness." For it has been with the advent of the 7000X phase-contrast video-enhanced computerized imaging system that the systemic invasion of such substances as candida, mycoplasmas, and pleomorphic or "L-forms" (as observed in the blood) may be established. Such microscopy also provides a tool with which to observe the elimination of fungi and bacteria and—with confirmatory electron microscopy—the elimination of viruses. This new dimension in microscopic observation allows the detection of the so-called "L-forms" (pleomorphic forms) which have long puzzled science. The explosive overgrowth of the latter in the body is now being recognized as a virtual market for allergies, sensitivities, and immune depression.

Research on Dioxychlor and its effects is in alignment with the concept of oxidology—the study of reactive oxygen toxic species (ROTS) and their metabolism in health and disease—as enunciated by the Bradford Institute last year. Such research also places Dioxychlor as the major oxidant, of demonstrated effectiveness superior to hydrogen peroxide and ozone, both of which—as indicated below—may be seen as double-edged-sword oxidative therapies.

Universal Reactive Syndrome

The institute continues to find evidence that environmental disease—particularly the multiple-sensitivity condition generally denominated "universal reactor syndrome" (URS) almost always characterized by systemic candida and multiple allergies and sensitivities with increasing autoimmune disorders—is to a large extent iatrogenic in nature.

This is because one of the mechanisms that generate so-called "L-forms" is the use of antibiotics, particularly such broad-based spectrum ones as tetracycline, so that the short-term relief of infection provided by such agents is countered by a possible long-term negative: that is, the antibiotics may not be actually killing target bacteria but converting them to pleomorphic forms which may not only be reactivated at a later date but continue to produce toxins and lead to URS. The conversion of bacteria to such L-forms may thus provide relief of symptoms—but at the same time set the stage for later pathology.

Our continuing research indicates that there are two types of pleomorphic forms—reversible and irreversible. One of the primary mechanisms in activating reversible L-forms is the classic oxidative generation response, as in inflammation, antibody-antigen activity, the influenza viruses, and physical and psychological stress.

A classic example is the URS patient—an environmentally ill individual who may be sensitive to everything from hydrocarbons, pesticides and paint, to a wide spectrum of foods. In reality these sensitivities are initiating systemic ROTS ("free radical") substances which in turn activate pleomorphic forms and trigger a clinical crisis reaction which may be far more acute than the sensitivity which set it off.

The above problem is exacerbated by toxins produced by pleomorphic forms, which in turn inhibit the "mixed-function oxidase system," an enzyme complex responsible for detoxifying environmental chemicals, be they organic or inorganic. If the mixed-function oxidase system is blocked or seriously impaired, it leaves the body defenseless against such substances as environmental chemicals.

Indeed, a vicious cycle is set up along these lines.

Step One: Long-term (or even high-concentration, short-term) abuse of antibiotics, contraception pills, corticosteroids, "recreational" drugs, metal toxicity, etc., leads to a general lowering of the immune system.

Step Two: The general lowering of natural immunity leads to a proliferation of microbial infections which in turn are treated by more antibiotics and other drugs.

Step Three: As such infections are treated by antibiotic drugs, microbes convert to, and thus generate, pleomorphic forms. These relatively non-antigenic pleomorphic forms ("cell wall-deficient forms") essentially escape immune surveillance, are resistant to antibiotics, and are capable of existing in all tissues including blood.

Step Four: These new structures in turn produce toxins which, among other things, inhibit the mixed-function oxidase system, the body's primary defense against environmental chemicals.

Step Five: The patient, now essentially defenseless against such chemicals, some of them carcinogenic, becomes hypersensitive to them. These new invaders further depress the immune system.

The result of this five-step biochemical process is the Universal Reactor Syndrome—a situation in which patients increasingly become sensitive to virtually everything in their environment, ranging from actual industrial chemicals to simple foods, and spanning the gamut from reactions to temperature and fluids to the clothing they wear or the sheets on which they sleep. URS becomes a traumatized daily struggle in which an already depressed immune system is constantly turning against itself. The result may be lethal in many cases, but even when not lethal is an unrelenting daily torture.

The Breakthrough of Dioxychlor

Dioxychlor represents a major breakthrough in the eradication of the pleomorphic or "L-forms" whose proliferation is so key to the development of URS. And the improved microscopy allows for the detection of such items in the scenario as system-wide L-forms and mycoplasmas.

Continuing clinical research at Bradford Research Institute, Mexico, has indicated a dramatic reduction in the reactions to all sensitivities through the elimination of systemic pleomorphic forms with Dioxychlor. We have been able not only to reverse URS clinically but—at least in terms of preliminary research—to have an equally impressive response in amyotrophic lateral sclerosis (ALS). This early research suggests a close tie between the symptomatology of ALS and L-form concentrations.

In many URS patients we also find a significant infection of mycoplasmas—the smallest of the living microorganisms—which are cell wall-deficient structures ranging in diameter from .1 to .5 microns and characterized by a void in the center. The membranes of these forms have receptors for specific human tissues and are prodigious producers of hydrogen peroxide. There are numerous species of mycoplasmas and many are named after the pathologies with which they are associated—for example, pulmonary, neurological, and arthritis mycoplasmas. Mycoplasmas have been destroyed in vivo by Dioxychlor, a fact which may in part account for the dramatic decrease in symptoms of the Universal Reactor Syndrome.

In vitro research indicates the destruction of pseudomonas and the earlier stated viruses within seconds and at low concentrations. *Candida albicans* and Epstein-Barr in vitro tests indicated destruction of the offending structures within seconds at a level of .75 parts per million. Current clinical research suggests such activity is duplicated in vivo.

The Background

Bradford Research Institute, noting that the natural mechanism of action of white blood cells in killing infectious agents is the production of highly active forms of oxygen—namely, the ROTS family—has further described certain inorganic oxidants which also provide active oxygen and mimic the natural activity of white blood cells. These substances include various halogens (chlorine, bromine, iodine) which act as carriers of an active form of oxygen which is later released. For various reasons related to low toxicity, Dioxychlor is the preferred member of this group to be used clinically. Indeed, the potency of the bound oxygen is demonstrated by realizing that Dioxychlor is highly effective at concentrations less than 1 part per million (ppm) that permit it to be used homeopathically.

The use of Dioxychlor as a substance dates back to World War I, when it was used by the Western powers to save the lives of soldiers with infections, particularly gangrene. It has since been found to have a multiplicity of uses which, at first glance, seem unrelated and with no apparent biochemical explanation.

In terms of fungicide use, it is noted that one antifungal agent in common use (nystatin) leads, with prolonged usage, to the development of resistance to the drug and continued symptoms. The mechanism of action of Dioxychlor is related to biochemical processes within the fungus which are so basic to survival that resistance is impossible; as a result, no new resistant strains develop from the use of Dioxychlor, unlike with other fungicides.

Dioxychlor is an inorganic compound composed of chlorine and two atoms of nascent oxygen covalently bonded. It is the chemical property of Dioxychlor which makes possible the release of nascent oxygen upon decomposition during its action as an oxidizing agent, leaving a non-toxic chloride residue. Certain aspects of the cellular immune system (specific white blood cells) utilize other mechanisms in the generation of highly reactive oxygen derivatives for the purpose of combating the invasion of foreign organisms. Without these protective mechanisms provided by the immune system involving oxygen derivatives, the ability to fight environmental chemicals as well as infection is blocked.

The immune system of many persons, particularly the elderly, is deficient in the ability to provide these highly reactive oxygen derivatives so necessary for attacking the great variety of viral, fungal, and bacterial invaders that are continually bombarding the human body. Those who are improperly equipped for fighting these invaders become easy targets for the many diseases they produce, with accompanying and sometimes bizarre symptoms.

The use of Dioxychlor assists the natural protective mechanisms of the body in counteracting these infectious agents which, if not adequately neutralized, will most certainly lead to disease.

Dioxychlor in pure form (anhydrous) is a liquid at 0°C having a deep red color. When mixed with water and at high dilution it is colorless.

Bohr atomic models indicate a "coordinate covalent" bond, but in this bond both electrons are contributed by one of the atoms (chlorine) and none by the other. In the covalent bond one electron is contributed by each of the atoms forming the bond.

When Dioxychlor reacts as an oxidizing agent, the oxygen atom first binds to a single atom (the one being oxidized) and then is dissociated from chlorine. An electron is then given up to chlorine forming the chloride ion. When one realizes that there are 5.3 g of chlorine ion per liter of human plasma, it becomes obvious that the small amount of chloride generated through the use of Dioxychlor is negligible.

Other Cytotoxic Oxidizing Agents Used Clinically

Dioxychlor is not the only oxidizing agent in clinical use. Another agent also providing active oxygen is hydrogen peroxide, which has been used in the treatment of arthritis, cancer, and other metabolic diseases. Hydrogen peroxide is commercially available in low concentrations for the treatment of topical microbial infections.

Ozone is being used both in Europe and at the American Biologics Hospital in Mexico to treat various diseases including cancer, blood coagulation disorders, and liver diseases, among others.

It is a developing precept of oxidology that the success of oxidative therapies depends on the type used, the concentration of the oxidant, and the target of use. For example, hydrogen peroxide may be used effectively as an antiviral sterilizing agent orally and topically. If hydrogen peroxide is used intravenously, great caution should be exercised since, among other things, cancer cells produce prodigious quantities of hydrogen peroxide and the IV administration of this substance may induce cancer to proliferate. This is not true, for example, of either ozone or Dioxychlor.

Ozone is a powerful oxidant which can be used effectively at the right concentration, time, and place—for example, as an intratumoral therapy in cancer or in the ozonation of blood to oxidize it and destroy potentially harmful viruses. But any administrative route which increases oxidative processes in the lung is injurious and should be handled with great care; hence the caveat on intravenous ozone administration.

Dioxychlor is currently used as a topical gel ("C2"—complexed with carboners), or as homeopathic drops ("C3"), or as a cryogenically purified intravenous infusion material ("C4").

Cytoxicity of Dioxychlor

Proof that Dioxychlor is cytotoxic to bacteria, fungus, and virus clinically is shown by data indicating its effectiveness as a disinfectant (outside the body).

Dioxychlor has been found to inactivate the organism causing Legionnaire's Disease (Legionella pneumophila).

The chemically related compound sodium periodate (NaIO) inhibited the virulence, decreased the respiration of, and increased the sensitivity to, phagocytosis of the common pathogen Listeria monocytogenes.

A germicidal solution was developed containing Dioxychlor at an acid pH (lactic acid). The solution gave complete kill of *Staphylococcus aureus*, pseudomonas, and *Candida albicans* spores within 10 minutes. If used in a ultrasound cleaning device, complete killing occurred in less than five minutes.

The bacterial virus f2 was rapidly inactivated with Dioxychlor. At pH 5-9 only GMP (guanosine monophosphate) reacted, while the amino acids cystine, tryptophan, and tryosine reacted rapidly.

Dioxychlor applied to polio virus separated the RNA from the protein coat (capsid). Dioxychlor reacted with the capsid protein and prevented the absorption, penetration, and normal uncoating of the virus. It also reacted with the viral RNA and impaired the ability of the nucleic acid to act as a template for replication.

Quote from
Leon Chaitow, N.D., D.O.

Leon Chaitow, N.D., D.O., of London, England, reports that the presence of parasites in many patients can make candidiasis very difficult to treat, and that parasite infestation encourages yeast overgrowth. When treatment results for candidiasis are poor, Dr. Chaitow recommends testing for coincidental parasitic infection. Before treatment for candidiasis, all parasitic infections must first be successfully treated. Researchers believe that candidiasis can become resistant to treatment because of parasites such as Giardia lamblia, amoebas, nematodes, and cestodes.

Parasites can be identified by means of blood, urine, and fecal testing as well as electroacupuncture biofeedback. According to Dr. Chaitow, this method is also useful for revealing how well the body will tolerate any medications which may be prescribed.

To get rid of identified parasites, Dr. Chaitow advises pursuing a comprehensive herbal medicine approach, rather than medication. "In many cases, antiparasitic prescriptive drugs have not proved to be lastingly effective," he points out. "They may diminish symptoms for one or two months, but the symptoms later return with full force." Parasites can be fought with high dosage probiotic substances such as acidophilus, bifidobacteria, and Lactobacillus bulgaricus. Treatment may last from eight to twelve weeks. Dr. Chaitow reports an 80 percent success rate in cases of seriously ill people afflicted with parasites and yeast overgrowth using this method.

—*Alternative Medicine*
compiled by the Burton Goldberg Group

8

Eight-Week Candida Overgrowth Elimination Program

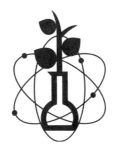

Required Products

Each product is designed to give a specific result. Do not make any substitutions. See page 291 for order form.

Arizona Natural Garlic	*Antifungal and blood purifier*
Caprystatin	*Antifungal for lower bowel, time-released*
Intestinal Cleanser	*Bulking agent to help clean out candida overgrowth*
Coenzyme Q10	*For strengthening the immune system*
DDS Acidophilus	*Restores friendly bacteria (always refrigerate)*
Kaprycidin-A	*Antifungal for stomach and small intestine*
Immuno-Quest	*For strengthening the immune system*
Natur-Earth	*Soil-based organism, antifungal*
Orithrush-D	*Gargle antifungal from mouth to stomach*
Pau D'Arco Tea	*Antifungal and immune builder*
Travacid X	*Digestive aid, time released HCl*
Dioxychlor DC3	*Antifungal/antiviral*
Latero Flora	*Antipathogen/antifungal*
OXY-OXC	*Oxygen therapy*

Candida Die-Off Reactions

During the eight-week program, it is not uncommon to experience symptoms attributed to the die-off reaction of the candida. These symptoms include feeling tired, spacey, dizzy and apathetic; or you may experience nausea, flu-like symptoms or a goopy sick feeling, muscular aches and pains, skin rashes, headaches, abdominal bloating, rectal itching, irritability, depression, food cravings, and difficulty in sleeping.

You can relieve some of these symptoms by getting plenty of rest at night, exercising, drinking at least eight glasses of water daily, eating regularly, and keeping snacks available throughout the day. Eating extra protein can also help relieve fatigue.

If you feel overly ill, you should stop the Caprystatin, Kaprycidin-A, and Orithrush-D gargle, but continue the other products until you feel better—usually one or two days. Then continue with the program where you left off.

Colon Therapy Recommendation

You should have one colon cleansing each week or as often as needed during the eight-week program. Bring one quart of Pau D'Arco Tea with you for colon cleansing, which will help to relieve candida die-off symptoms. If you are unable to locate a qualified colon therapist in your area, you should administer frequent enemas.

Colonic . . . A Gentle Irrigation for Your Colon

Why should I take a colonic?

The colon's main function is the elimination of the body's waste. We experience health and well-being when the colon is clean and normal. When the colon is sluggish, hardened feces lodge in the pockets of the colon walls, resulting in constipation. This hardened matter then obstructs the muscular contractions (peristalsis), reducing the colon's ability to properly evacuate. This waste buildup of many months or years may weigh as much as 15 pounds, causing a distended and abnormally shaped colon. The clogged colon then interferes with final absorption and digestion of food, depriving the body of necessary nutrients. This results in fermentation and putrefaction of undigested food, which create poisons. These poisons are reabsorbed into the bloodstream and are carried to every part of the body causing a tired and listless feeling. The brain and nervous system become toxic, causing depression and irritability; the lungs create foul breath and stressful breathing; the digestive organs create skin problems and sallow complexion; and the joints may become stiff and painful due to toxic deposits.

Can I be constipated even if I have 1, 2, or 3 bowel movements a day?

Yes. Accumulated wastes, mucous, and gas in the colon may inhibit its natural peristaltic action, resulting in incomplete—though frequent—bowel movements.

What is a colon irrigation?

A colon irrigation is the gradual and gentle introduction of warm, purified water into the colon to help stimulate its natural peristalsis. The colon irrigation, or colonic, tickles the colon walls with water, which helps the colon to release impacted wastes and mucous. Before starting the procedure, the therapist gently inserts into the rectum a sterile, disposable speculum attached to a hose leading to the colonic machine. The client reclines comfortably on his/her back during the course of the treatment, while warm, purified water is slowly administered. After the colon has been sufficiently stimulated, the therapist releases the water pressure. The water and wastes from the colon pass through the hose into the machine's waste drain, and fresh water is again introduced into the colon. The gentle water flow is always under the direct control of the therapist, who repeats the process of fills and releases for 40-50 minutes.

How many times do I need to take a colonic?

Often the waste is so hard and deeply lodged in the colon that a series of colonics may be necessary to sufficiently soften and loosen it. Colonics also stimulate the liver, kidney, and lymph system to dump toxins. The number of treatments varies with each individual and his/her condition. Your therapist can best advise you regarding this.

Are colonics habit-forming?

No. The purpose of cleansing the colon is to allow it to relax and rejuvenate and promote better peristalsis. The colon cannot heal when it is constantly working to get rid of accumulated wastes, gases, and poisons.

Won't colonics damage the normal intestinal flora?

Accumulation of encrusted feces in the colon makes it impossible for the glands to produce the necessary intestinal flora, resulting in increased constipation. Cleansing the colon helps bring the acid-alkaline ratio back into balance, allowing friendly bacteria to thrive, while inhibiting disease-causing organisms. You can assist the body in this process by orally taking acidophilus to reintroduce friendly bacteria into the colon.

Dietary Instructions

Foods Not Allowed

Beverages: Alcoholic products such as beer, wine, champagne, saki, hard liquor, and liqueurs. Fruit juices, sodas, and other beverages containing natural or artificial sweeteners. All carbonated beverages.

Sugar Products: Simple sugars such as sucrose, maltose, dextrose, galactose, and fructose. Refined sugars (junk sugars) such as white, brown, and raw sugar. Syrups such as molasses, sorghum, maple syrup, and honey. Sugar foods such as candy, chocolate, cakes, pies, cookies, ice cream, sherbet, and any foods with artificial sweeteners.

Fruits: Fresh, dried, frozen, and canned fruits.

Yeast Products: Bread, crackers, brewer's yeast, natural B vitamins, and any products with yeast added (examine labels for vitamin and mineral yeast-based ingredients).

Fermented and Mold Foods: Cheeses, cultured dairy products, buttermilk, sour cream, mushrooms, cider, malts, tofu, soy sauce, miso, pickled foods, vinegar, mustard, catsup, relish, and other condiments made with vinegar.

Peanuts: Peanut butter and peanut products.

Hard Fats: Fats that stay solid at room temperature such as margarine, shortening, and hydrogenated oils.

Processed Meats: Meats and fish that are cured, dried, breaded, pickled, or smoked, such as ham, bacon, corned beef, pastrami, salami, hot dogs, lunch meats, and sausages.

Refined Foods: White flour and white rice.

Tubers: Sweet potatoes, white potatoes, and yams.

Foods Allowed

Beverages: Water (preferably purified), water flavored with lemon juice, herbal teas (no caffeine), decaffeinated beverages, Pero or other grain beverages, and almond milk.

Breakfast Foods: Unsweetened hot cereal, 7-grain, rice flakes, oatmeal, and oat bran.

Carbohydrates: Almonds, sunflower seeds, pumpkin seeds, and Brazil nuts, but no other kinds of nuts or seeds. Puffed rice cakes, legumes, beans, peas, lentils, corn, buckwheat, soybeans, soya products, grains, millet, and brown rice. Any of these may be ground or combined to make recipes such as noodles, crackers, and breads, as long as no yeast or sugar is added.

Protein: Preferably chicken and fish; however, lean beef, lamb, and veal are acceptable. Moderate use of eggs.

Vegetables: All kinds of cooked and raw vegetables. Frozen vegetables are acceptable, but check labels to be sure they do not contain sugar, vinegar, or additives.

Dairy: Moderate amounts of plain low-fat yogurt, low-fat milk and butter, preferably unsalted raw butter.

Condiments: Spices, herbs, and sea salt. Dressings made without vinegar such as oil and lemon juice or homemade mayonnaise.

Oils: Moderate use of cold-pressed olive oil (refrigerate), sesame oil, almond oil, and tahini.

Eight-Week Candida Overgrowth Elimination Program Schedule and Dosage

Week One

Date Started: _____ Date Completed: _____

Natur-Earth	2 *upon arising with water only*	
Latero Flora	2 *upon arising with water only*	*Take these 5 products at the same time*
DDS Acidophilus	2 *upon arising with water only*	
Travacid X	1 *upon arising with water only*	
OXY-OXC	4 *upon arising with water only*	

Dioxychlor DC3   *10 drops under tongue twice daily; hold for 3 minutes, then swallow*

Travacid X	1 *before lunch and dinner*	
Caprystatin	1 *twice daily before meals*	
Coenzyme Q10	1 *twice daily before meals*	*Take these 6 products at the same time before meals*
Arizona Natural Garlic	3 *twice daily before meals*	
Intestinal Cleanser	2 *twice daily before meals*	
Immuno-Quest	2 *twice daily before meals*	

Pau D'Arco Tea   *No more than 6 oz. daily*
Directions: Add 1 heaping tablespoon Pau D'Arco Tea to 4 cups boiling water. Simmer 20 minutes. Strain and refrigerate. Drink either hot or cold.

Week Two

Date Started: _____ Date Completed: _____

Take all products as in the first week, with the following change:
Caprystatin   2 *twice daily before meals*

Week Three

Date Started:_____ Date Completed:_____

Take all products as in the first week, with the following change:
Caprystatin   3 *twice daily before meals*

Week Four

Date Started:_____ Date Completed:_____

Take all products as in the first week, with the following changes:
Caprystatin   3 *twice daily before meals*
Kaprycidin-A   1 *twice daily before meals*

Week Five

Date Started:_____ Date Completed:_____

Take all products as in the first week, with the following changes:
Latero Flora   1 *upon arising with water only*
Caprystatin   3 *twice daily before meals*
Kaprycidin-A   2 *twice daily before meals*

Week Six

Date Started:_____ Date Completed:_____

Take all products as in the first week, with the following changes:
Latero Flora   1 *upon arising with water only*
Caprystatin   3 *twice daily before meals*
Kaprycidin-A   3 *twice daily before meals*

Week Seven

Date Started:_____ Date Completed:_____

Take all products as in the first week, with the following changes:

Latero Flora	*1 upon arising with water only*
Caprystatin	*3 twice daily before meals*
Kaprycidin-A	*3 twice daily before meals*
Orithrush-D Gargle	*Mix 1 part with 20 parts water (no refrigeration necessary); gargle and then swallow one mouthful of this mixture twice daily.*

Week eight

Date Started:_____ Date Completed:_____

Take all products as in the seventh week.

Congratulations!

You have completed the Candida Overgrowth Elimination Program! Now you should continue with the instructions on the following pages.

Post-Program Maintenance

1. After completing the eight-week program, discontinue the following products:
   Caprystatin, Kaprycidin-A, and Orithrush-D Gargle.
2. You will have some other products remaining after the eighth week. Finish the remainder of the following products as follows:
   Intestinal Cleanser   *2 twice daily before meals*
   Arizona Natural-Garlic   *3 twice daily before meals*
3. Continue to take the following products for 3 months as follows:

Natur-Earth	*2 upon arising with water only*
DDS Acidophilus	*2 upon arising with water only*
Travacid X	*1 upon arising with water only, and 1 before lunch and dinner*
Latero Flora	*1 upon arising with water only*
OXY-OXC	*4 upon arising with water only*
Dioxychlor DC$_3$	*5 drops under tongue twice daily; hold 3 minutes, then swallow*
Coenzyme Q10	*1 twice daily before meals*
Immuno-Quest	*2 twice daily before meals*
Pau D'Arco Tea	*No more than 1 cup daily*

4. Slowly add restricted foods back into your diet. For the first few days, only add fermented foods. For the next few days add sweet foods, such as fruits, juices, and honey. Try to avoid all alcoholic beverages for 30 days.
   If you experience a recurrence of symptoms, return to the restricted diet for 30 days and take three Caprystatin twice daily before meals in addition to the products in instruction 3 above.
5. Avoid commercial meats, commercially-raised chicken, and commercial eggs from caged chickens, since they contain antibiotics, stimulants, growth hormones, and

pesticides. Your local health food store should have organic meat, organic chicken (such as Rocky Road chicken), and eggs that are free of these chemicals. You can purchase organic beef from Coleman's Beef, 707 East 50th Street, Denver, CO 80216. Choose wisely, ask questions, and don't settle for less than clean, chemical-free food.

6. At some future time due to illness, you may be required to take an antibiotic. After you have completed the full cycle of the medication, take two DDS Acidophilus capsules daily (with water only upon arising) to rebuild your intestinal flora. This will help you avoid any future candida yeast overgrowth.

Letters from Satisfied Clients

February 6, 1992

Dear Stanley:
Thank you so much for treating my problem. I have not had any more trouble with candida since I took your treatment.
I am so grateful to you for curing my disease.
I have no rash, no allergic reactions to sugar or yeast foods and my energy is back—all thanks to you. I am not taking any nystatin either.

Wishing you all the best,
Carol Heald

June 22, 1994

To whom it may concern:
As a 27-year employee of a major airline, I found myself exposed, through travel to many exotic ports, to a frightening array of parasitic creatures. For 6 years, I found out the full extent of what traditional medicine did not know. I almost accepted as normal the fatigue, infections, antibiotics, allergies, yeast problems and indigestion that I regularly experienced. Finally, a year ago, I visited Stan Weinberger's Healing Within clinic and took the full parasitic treatment. This was followed by the candida program. I now have a major reduction of all the above-mentioned problems, and the progress is continuing. And while certain portions of the program have required strict dietary restrictions and some discipline, the results are without question worth every effort.

Sincerely,
Loni Blissard
Honolulu, Hawaii

March 24, 1995

Dear Stanley:

I am writing this letter to say thank you for your book, Healing Within: The Complete Guide to Colon Health, *and for what has happened in my life as a result of reading it.*

For years, I have been trying to get to the bottom of why I never felt well. In recent years, I have had a lot of aches and pains and an awful time with constipation and gas and being tired. I tried different diets and was diagnosed once for yeast, but nothing ever seemed to work to make me feel better. I have been to M.D.s, Naturopaths, Health Food Stores, had Cytotoxic Testing, etc. I was always full of gas and either constipated or with diarrhea (constipation has been a longstanding problem with me). Also, I had a lot of tension in my neck muscles and shoulders and low back. I had massage treatments for relief and was at the chiropractor a lot, but nothing ever cleared up any of this. I was really at the end of my rope. But at one point, I felt deep down that somehow when my husband and I moved to the Cape, the Lord was going to help me find the solution to all this chronic stuff.

My daughter is an occupational therapist and massage therapist and she suggested that I try acupuncture for the constipation. But first I saw a nutritionist, Marcia Sloane, at the Cape Cod Center for Holistic Medicine. That was the beginning of the great changes in my health/life.

Marcia told me that I had classic candida symptoms and she started me on a program of diet and supplements. Within three days I noticed a change for the better with my gut/digestion. As the months passed, however, the constipation never really got better. Marcia could not under-

stand it, so we tried acupuncture, but it did not help, nor did the Chinese herbs. I asked Marcia if she thought colonics might help. She said it was certainly worth a try, so I had a treatment. Nothing much changed, but I did feel better in my gut initially.

My husband and I then went to England for six months and I had 13 more colonic treatments and all of the aches and pains and muscle tension went away! I was eating a food-combining diet, losing some weight, and having much more energy. The colonic therapist was also muscle testing me, which indicated that the candida was definitely getting better and I did not show any parasites.

When we came home from England, I continued to feel good and was sticking to the diet, and continued the colonics. But when I went back for a check on the yeast, it was still not as good as it should be. It was very defeating to me that the yeast was still there and I just couldn't understand why this thing can't be licked the way other things can be. Why does yeast so easily come back with the slightest going off the diet?

At this point, I asked Connie Jones, who gave me a copy of your book, whether any of her clients had ever tried your Candida Overgrowth Elimination Program. She said they had, and that they had good results. She suggested I call you and order it.

I did call you, and after explaining my situation, you said that you had found that when candida is so insidious, it may not be the underlying problem. That was very interesting, because so many of my other problems had candida as the underlying cause and now I was hearing there could be an underlying cause for the candida! Sort of like layers of an onion . . . You suggested that I do the Parasite Elimination Program, which I did. I will admit that I was not totally strict with the candida type diet you recommended, but I stuck pretty much to it.

CHAPTER 8

To make a long story short, I was angry for the first few weeks, and my stomach was as hard as a rock. I knew something was going on. I did call you and you said those were normal kinds of reactions because I was ingesting poison, not nutrients. When I went for a colonic, my right side was extremely sore and tender, which it had never been before, and Connie said that was a very good sign because that is where the parasites like to live.

Shortly before I completed the Parasite Elimination Program, I asked the nutritionist to muscle test me for yeast. She did a lot of testing and when she was done, she said, "What have you been doing? There is no sign of yeast at all, not even a subtle sign!"

I cannot tell you how happy I was. Praise the Lord! Then I told her about the Parasite Elimination Program I had been doing and that this might be an answer for others who have chronic yeast. As I said earlier, after we had moved to the Cape, I really felt that somehow the Lord was going to heal me of the constipation and other symptoms. I think that all I have been through and all my searching was with His help and that somehow this experience of mine may help others down the road. What I want to say is a very big thank you to you, Stanley, for your help.

My constipation problem is getting better too, as I still take extra herbs to stay regular, but now that I have started the Oxy-Oxc, I am taking less of them and think that the Oxy-Oxc is helping. Connie had said that part of my problem may be genetic, which is possible, because my mother and sister have the same problem.

In closing, I want to say that it is a whole new life healthwise for me and even mentally, as I am beginning to remember things much more quickly and just have more energy. I exercise every day and stay up later and do more than I have in a long time. God bless you in your *work and for getting the word out. I hope all the yeast doctors who are treating people will not discount the parasite connection in all of this, but see it as another cause.*

Sincerely and gratefully,
Laura Lee W.
(last name witheld by request)

9

Parasites: An Epidemic in Disguise

THE FAR SIDE

By GARY LARSON

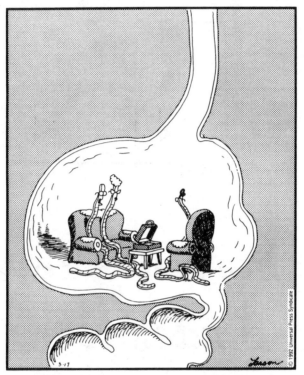

"Well, I'm not sure if we can afford stomach
insurance — right now we're trying to put the kids
through the small intestine."

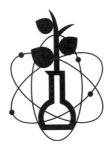

Parasites: An Epidemic in Disguise

The first major nationwide survey of parasitic diseases has revealed that one in every six people studied has one or more parasites living somewhere in his or her body.
—Ronald Kotulak

A parasite epidemic in America? You must be joking! This is a clean, well-fed nation—parasites are only a serious problem in Third World countries . . . aren't they?

This attitude—that Americans are too clean, too civilized, too well-fed and too well-educated for parasites to be a serious problem—is surprisingly prevalent. Yet, there are about 300 types of parasites thriving in America today, including pinworms, tapeworms, hookworms, ringworms, whipworms, roundworms and *Giardia lamblia*. In fact, the microscopic parasite, Giardia, has infected the waterways in many of our nation's parks. Parasites know no national boundaries. They are oblivious to your income, your nationality, your age and your beliefs. More than 80 percent of the world's population is infected with parasites, which can range in size from microscopic to 20 feet in length. According to the Center for Disease Control, virtually every known parasitic disease has been diagnosed in the United States!

Most people know you can get tapeworms from eating under-cooked pork. But did you know you can get parasites from eating a rare steak? Or from just shaking hands with an infected person? Or from playing with your pet? You might even get parasites from your children—who picked up the little freeloaders from their friends at school. You can also get parasites from eating raw vegetables on which the tiny parasite eggs are laid. Sex also spreads parasites: they are more easily passed than venereal diseases through sexual practices.

The two major factors that make an epidemic of parasites possible are: 1) lack of sanitation; and 2) colons which are clogged and impacted from years of improper eating habits, providing a warm and well-fed breeding ground for worms and parasites to proliferate.

You may have very clean habits in your own kitchen, but do you eat out in restaurants? Many restaurants and food handlers are shockingly negligent in the most basic sanitation practices.

And how aware are you about the health of your intestinal tract? Parasites usually live in the intestinal tract, where they look forward to a steady diet of their favorite foods: sugar-laden desserts, and fried, processed, and other junk foods. Even if you have a healthy, well-balanced diet, once your system is infected with parasites, you are at their mercy. They breed happily, growing fat and sassy stealing your nutrition, drinking your blood, and fouling your system with their wastes, which are reabsorbed into your bloodstream and carried to all parts of your body. Parasites take a heavy toll on the immune system and its function.

Symptoms of parasitic infestation run a wide range. Roundworms cause fever, cough, and intestinal problems. Hookworms cause anemia, abdominal pain, diarrhea, apathy, malnutrition, and even under-development in children. Whipworms cause abdominal pain and diarrhea.

The fecal matter from a single tapeworm can make humans ill. The worms may become so numerous as to cause intestinal obstruction as well as gas and intestinal distress. Tapeworm eggs in the liver can be mistaken for cancer and chemotherapy may be administered. The chemo will kill the eggs, but may also harm the patient.

Bloodflukes make lesions in the lungs and cause hemorrhages under the skin. They are often found in AIDS patients. Protozoa, such as amoeba, do not suck blood like the hookworm and others do, but these creatures cause arthritis-like pains or leukemia-like symptoms, and generally weaken the entire system.

Giardia lamblia, a protozoan parasite resembling the single-celled amoeba, is the most prevalent parasite in the U.S. today and is considered the number one cause of waterborne disease in the country. Giardia causes diarrhea, weakness, weight loss, abdominal cramps, nausea, belching and fever. The tiny parasites can coat the inside lining of the small intestine and prevent the lining from absorbing nutrients from food.

The multitude of different symptoms caused by parasites can be baffling to many doctors, who receive little training in diagnosing and treating parasitic infections. Unless people have major symptoms, doctors often misdiagnose cases as bacterial infections, but unfortunately, antibiotics have no effect on most parasites.

Colon cleansing (colonics) can go a long way toward eliminating parasites and accumulated, impacted wastes in the large intestine. These wastes can be caused by eating the wrong kinds of foods, drinking too little liquid, lack of exercise, improper combination of foods, emotional distress, and weak muscle tone of the colon. Removal of these wastes by colon cleansing—wherein the colon is flushed with filtered water through a series of fills and releases—results in a renewed sense of health, vitality, and energy in the individual's entire system.

But to remove all the parasites which may be living in the colon, small intestine, blood stream and many organs of the body, it is essential to embark upon an effective parasite elimination program, in conjunction with colon cleansings.

Parasites can be destroyed harmlessly without injury to the

body and without dangerous drugs by following the *Healing Within* 60-Day Parasite Elimination Program. This program starts with the "parasite killer" colon complements: Gozarte with Neo-Pararte; or, for persons who also have a candida problem, Gozarte with Udarte. Pasaloc and Padapco are a good choice if the individual is taking a lot of antioxidants and can't reduce them for the 60-day period. Pasaloc and Padapco are also a good choice if worms are present. Finally, K-Min, Black Walnut Tincture, Castor Oil Capsules, *Healing Within* Intestinal Cleanser and Latero Flora are included in all programs. The immune system is strengthened by the use of Echinacea, Shitake Mushroom Capsules and DDS Acidophilus. Finally, the addition of Intestinalis Herbal Cleanser at the end of the *Healing Within* Parasite Elimination Program protects the intestinal tract from reinfestation. These products will destroy almost every parasite known to humankind.

Gozarte, Udarte, Neo-Pararte, Pasaloc, and Padapco are powerful herbal combinations organically grown in the rain forests of Columbia. K-Min is a balance of mined elements that will, by ionization, rip worms apart. Since parasites rarely pass out of the body whole (and antibiotics have no effect on them), K-Min was devised to rip them up. Black Walnut Tincture, an herbal fluid, is very effective against parasites that may make their way into the bloodstream and to other organs of the body. In fact, K-Min and Black Walnut Tincture can be given to animals to rid them of parasites.

Good old-fashioned castor oil is not a mineral oil; it is the oil of the castor plant bean and it has been known as a potent laxative for centuries. Castor oil lubricates the walls of the colon and helps loosen the hardened, impacted waste materials. Thanks to modern science, you can now take this cathartic and intestinal-wall lubricant without the unpleasant taste by ingesting frozen Castor Oil Capsules. The frozen capsules pass through the stomach and do not dissolve until they reach the small intestine, where they do the most good.

Healing Within Intestinal Cleanser contains gentian, golden seal, buckthorn, rhubarb root, cascara sagrada, and aloe vera, all well calculated and delicately balanced in proportions essential for the success of the cleanser and detoxifier. This grouping pulls mucous, detoxifies, heals, acts as a diuretic, activates flushing of the liver and production of bile, and improves intestinal peristalsis.

Latero Flora (Bacillus laterosporus—B.O.D. strain) normalizes the flora in the human digestive tract, aids in digestion and toxin elimination, and discourages the growth of yeast, fungi, and other pathogenic micro-organisms. Latero Flora is extremely effective for individuals with gastrointestinal disturbances, food allergies, and candidiasis hypersensitivity syndrome. No other product in existence is as effective as Latero Flora in restoring the original, desirable bacterial balance to the intestines, thus aiding in resolving many immuno-suppressed conditions.

The *Healing Within* Parasite Elimination Program is a safe, non-toxic, natural and effective method of removing parasites from the body. The combination of herbs provides the greatest strength and efficacy of any known parasite elimination products in the world. Where others have failed, these products have succeeded.

In conjunction with the program, it is also highly advisable to have colon cleansings once a week to assist in the removal of live and dead parasites and accumulated colon wastes. If colon cleansings are not available, several enemas a week are essential.

Completing the program will not necessarily be easy. Work and dedication are required, but the rewards may be greater than you think. The results of the *Healing Within* Parasite Elimination Program and colon cleansings can include elimination of painful and uncomfortable symptoms, a stronger immune system, a greater sense of vitality and well-being, clearer thinking and improved memory, and an increased zest for life. Remember, the old adage, "Health, wealth and happiness" always begins with health!

Worms Outrank Cancer as Man's Deadliest Enemy

by Dolly Katz

Every year, the American Cancer Society publishes the names of famous people, such as Duke Ellington and Jack Benny, who have died of cancer. This is done, the society says, as "a dramatic reminder of the full dimensions of cancer's human devastation."

When Abdel Halim Hafez, the most popular singer in the Arab world, died last year, his name did not appear on any list, although the disease that killed him causes more human devastation than cancer does. Hafez, 46, died from complications of schistosomiasis, an infection of parasitic worms that live in the intestines. Worldwide, an estimated 258 million people—the equivalent of the entire U.S. population—are infected with this disease.

And the schistosomiasis worm is only one of many parasites, ranging in size from microscopic single-celled animals to foot-long roundworms, which annually kill many more people than cancer does. The diseases they cause are as well known as malaria and as obscure as kala-azar, which particularly affects children and is 90 percent fatal if untreated.

One of every four people in the world is infected by roundworms, which cause fever, cough, and intestinal problems. A quarter of the world's people have hookworms, which can cause anemia and abdominal pain. A third of a billion people suffer from the abdominal pain and diarrhea caused by whipworms.

Not much research is being done on these diseases. The U.S. spends more than $800 million a year on cancer research. All the nations of the world combined spend less than one-twentieth that amount studying parasitic diseases. As a result, there are no vaccines against them, and many of them are difficult or impossible to treat. There is no known treatment, for instance, for Chagas' disease, a variant of African sleeping sickness that occurs in South and Central America.

But while these diseases occur predominately in underdeveloped countries, the U.S. is not immune to them. Just about every parasitic disease known has been diagnosed in the U.S. in the last few years: schistosomiasis, trichinosis, giardiasis, toxoplasmosis, African sleeping sickness.

Most, like malaria, are imported cases brought back by travelers. But a significant number are entrenched in parts of our environment, kept alive in the U.S. by person-to-person transmission.

Pinworms, for example, parasites that live in the lower intestine and rectum, are the most common parasitic infection of children in temperate countries. At least one in five children in the general population has pinworms; in institutions, the figure can go as high as 90 percent.

All this doesn't mean that Americans ought to add parasites to the long list of diseases we're supposed to worry about when we develop symptoms. But it's interesting and perhaps important to realize that to most of the world's people, cancer is as exotic a disease as sleeping sickness is to us.

Reprinted from *The Miami Herald,* June 25, 1978.

Parasites More Common than Believed, Study Says

by Ronald Kotulak

The first major nationwide survey of parasitic diseases has revealed that one in every six people studied has one or more parasites living somewhere in his or her body.

The prevalence of these parasitic stowaways, which range from microscopic organisms to 15-foot tapeworms, has come as a big surprise, especially to physicians who receive little training in diagnosing and treating parasitic infections.

"We think of this country as a highly sanitized country," Dr. Myron G. Schulz said, "but that is not necessarily true."

The large number of parasites, he said, means they are causing many diseases that baffle doctors.

"Many patients have experienced weeks of delay before the correct diagnosis was made and have been subjected to unnecessary laboratory tests, hospitalization, and even surgery," Shultz, director of the parasitic diseases division of the Centers for Disease Control (CDC) in Atlanta, warned in an editorial in the *Journal of the American Medical Association*.

He said that the presence of parasites also means that many Americans are not as "clean" as they thought they were.

"What concerns me is that somewhere along the line there has been a breakdown in sanitation measures and people have ingested contaminated food, water, or dirt," said Dr. Dennis Juranek, assistant chief of the CDC's parasitic diseases division.

The survey pinpointed four problems:

- A parasite that causes intestinal infections is sweeping across the country. Called *Giardia lamblia,* the parasite has now become the number one cause of waterborne disease in the nation.

- Tapeworm infections appear to have increased by 100 percent in the last ten years, an increase that may be linked to American's increasing fondness for raw or rare beef.

- Amebiasis, the most deadly of the parasites, continues to be a serious problem, with recent outbreaks in South Carolina. Between 1969 and 1973 there were 242 reported deaths from amebiasis, a microscopic organism usually passed from person to person.

- Illinois farmers are being plagued by a Balatidium parasite from pigs that causes intestinal infections in humans.

The survey involved examinations of 414,820 samples of feces in 1976. The examinations were performed by 570 public and private laboratories in all 50 states and the results sent to the CDC.

According to the survey, 15.6 percent of the specimens contained one or more parasites. About half these parasites are capable of causing disease.

The large number of parasitic infections discovered in the survey may not reflect the actual rate of infection in the general public, but it does reveal that the problem is much more widespread than most health professionals thought.

"I'm sure that this high infection rate comes as a surprise to those who never considered parasitic diseases to be a major problem in the U.S.," Dr. Juranek said.

The biggest problem uncovered in the survey was the high rate of infection with the Giardia parasite.

This parasite now appears to have spread to almost every state and is responsible for recent epidemics in upstate New York, Colorado, Washington, New Hampshire, and Wisconsin.

This bug, a protozoan parasite, is microscopic in size and resembles a single-celled amoeba. The parasite coats the inside lining of the small intestine and prevents the lining from absorbing nutrients from food.

Although not a killer, it causes illness characterized by diarrhea, weakness, weight loss, abdominal cramps, nausea, vomiting, belching, and fever.

Most cases are misdiagnosed as bacterial infections, but unfortunately antibiotics have no effect on the parasite, Dr. Juranek said. Two drugs are effective in curing Giardias: atabrine, an antimalarial agent, and metronidazole.

Hundreds of small water systems throughout the country that do not adequately purify water may be contaminated with the parasite, said Dr. John Hoff, an EPA research microbiologist.

Streams or watersheds may become contaminated through infected human sewage, and recent studies show that Giardia-infected beavers may also contaminate water sources.

Reprinted from *The Chicago Tribune Service.*

Parasites and AIDS

by Rev. Hanna Kroeger

AIDS (Acquired Immune Deficiency Syndrome) is not one disease in itself. Rather it is caused by the accumulation of several factors that weaken the immune system so drastically that the body is susceptible to many other diseases.

Parasites, such as hookworm and protozoa, are found in almost all carriers of AIDS. The most common type of hookworm found, Hydatoxi Lualba, is microscopic and can travel into the lung tissue making lesions. It also can be found in the brain, intestines, rectum, and intracutaneous tissue. It is the same microscopic disturbance that causes uremic poisoning during pregnancy.

Widespread protozoa, a freshwater parasite causing weakening of the entire system, is also found in AIDS carriers. Protozoa do not suck blood as the hookworm does, but make arthritis-like pains, leukemia symptoms, bleeding under the skin, and a host of other symptoms. Dr. Bingham, author of the book *Fight Back Against Arthritis*, states on page 52:

> Overall, it seems highly probable that various species of free-living protozoa are the etiological agent of collagene-anti-immune disease which show every graduation and combination with one another. They are not due to a single organism, but to a number of similar organisms. Such a parasitic infection would explain the urticaria asthma and easinophilia observed in many cases of collagene or auto-immune diseases.

Sometimes flukes and flatworms are found in the blood of AIDS sufferers. These bloodflukes make lesions in the lungs and hemorrhages under the skin.

Finally, *Candida albicans*, the hidden epidemic, is always found in AIDS victims. This fungus overgrowth can affect every organ and part of the body and is the worst of the fungi that attack the nervous system.

Reprinted by permission of Rev. Hanna Kroeger, 7075 Valmont Drive, Boulder, CO 80301.

Note: Although Dr. Louis Parrish reports only some success with his method of treatment in the following article, the *Healing Within Herbal Parasite Elimination Program* has a high success rate. Rarely does the herbal program have to be repeated, unless there is a reinfestation of parasites. Preventing a parasitic infestation is now possible thanks to a new herbal combination from Colombia called Consolar. Consolar sets up a barrier in the stomach against parasites and should be taken before eating meals in restaurants or when traveling. Refer to page 291 to order.   —S.W.

The Protozoal Syndrome

by Louis Parrish, M.D.

For almost two decades, I have been trying to raise medical and lay community awareness regarding a major health problem, infections of intestinal protozoa *Entamoeba histolytica* and *Giardia lamblia,* which alone or together are often devastating to the quality of a person's life. Although separate diseases, they have so much in common that I refer to them collectively as the Protozoal Syndrome.

The symptoms these organisms produce in humans are so varied, intermittent, and similar to other infections involving the immune system, that only relatively recently are they being recognized as a primary cause of generalized illness.

A Brief History

Intestinal parasites have existed since our evolution as homo sapiens, yet were only recognized as medical entities in the last 200 years. These protozoa may even have been a factor in Darwinian selection. Diarrheal diseases are a primary cause of infant mortality. Those with a strong immune system and better nutrition survive, but during their lives many may never recognize a normal bowel or realize their full energy potential. I have often wondered if the Latin siesta was not a cultural manifestation of unnatural lethargy caused by these organisms.

These prevalent, potentially disabling diseases, especially amoebic dysentery, became important diagnoses along with typhoid fever in the early 1900s. With the New Deal, work forces did a laudable job cleaning up the environment, setting standards to eliminate polluted water, and establishing public health centers. The incidence of Amoebiasis and Giardiasis was reduced during that time period, though never controlled. In the last five decades they have been on the rise due to world wars, peripatetic tourists, and most importantly, immigrant food handlers from endemic areas.

Millions Affected in U. S. A. Alone

Based on my experience, I estimate in the New York metropolitan area that 25 percent of the population is infected. Of these, 15 percent are asymptomatic, 25 percent have ignorable symptoms, 55 percent have a compromised quality of life, and 5 percent are disabled. Using a conversion factor of .1 among 258 million U.S. inhabitants, I feel confident in estimating that 7 million people are infected. In addition, virtually every sexually transmitted AIDS patient I have seen is, or has been, infected with Amoebiasis or Giardiasis.

Effects on the Immune System

A Giardia invasion of the duodenum and upper small intestine can significantly reduce production of Immunoglobulin A, the most important source of secretory antibodies. Furthermore, in relating an endemic outbreak of Amoebiasis two years prior to the outbreak of AIDS in San Francisco, researchers from the University of Virginia reported that amoebas can project an activated substance, a lectin, which ruptures the immune defense cells that have by ingestion inactivated the HIV virus. Freed into the bloodstream, they multiply and manifest their lethal potential. The implications of an amoebic infection on immune function are obvious and applicable to other viral infections.

Alarming Misconceptions

The medical establishment rests shamefully complacent with some alarming misconceptions about these diseases:

Misconception 1: These diseases exist only in tropical, unsanitary geographic areas.

- The fact is that there are other areas where the infections are alarmingly prevalent, with the U.S.A. having a high but unrecognized incidence. These pathogenic organisms thrive in areas as diverse as the cold rushing mountain streams and placid lakes of our national parks, which beavers and perhaps other animals have contaminated with their feces, to the sushi and salad bars of our metropolitan areas, transmitted by "fecal fingers" of food handlers, especially immigrants from countries where hand washing is not routine after a bowel evacuation.

- Recently at a large Manhattan hotel I asked the attendant in the men's room to count the number of people who entered the stalls and how many washed their hands when they came out. In a two-hour period 112 entered, but only 60 washed their hands. Assuming that 15 percent of those only urinated and were less likely to wash, 44 could have left with potentially contaminated hands. The bathroom was located at the site of a Health Convention! This anecdotal report reflects the insidious spread of these infections.

Misconception 2: These diseases are species specific, passed only from human to human.

- There is increasing evidence to challenge this assumption. Besides the wild animals that pollute the outdoor water supplies, pooper-scoopers, cat litter attendants, as well as parakeet owners, are all at risk of contracting the disease from their pets.

Misconception 3: An accurate diagnosis can be obtained from a single stool exam.

- Good parasitology teaches that one must get three

specimens. If they are negative and one is still clinically suspicious, get three to six more. Some authorities recommend treating all patients with a suggestive clinical presentation, even if no protozoa are found. Often a therapeutic trial is the best diagnostic procedure.

Misconception 4: Treatment with a single course of metronizadole-Flagyl is 90 percent effective.

• Fact: 25 years ago this may have been true. But the protozoa rapidly became resistant. Today the single course cure rate is less than 5 percent. Furthermore, approximately half of the patients treated with metronizadole complain of side effects, and 10 percent flatly refuse to take it ever again.

Symptoms

After 30 years' experience, I have divided the many symptoms of the Protozoal Syndrome into three categories:

Gastrointestinal: Oral thrush, indigestion, acid reflux, epigastric discomfort, malabsorption, gas, foul flatus, mucus sometimes blood-tinged, erratic and unpredictable bowel movements, urgency, weird stool formations—from explosive liquid diarrhea to prolonged periods of constipation and anal irritation.

Fatigue: Persistent tiredness, excessive yet unrefreshing sleep, lack of motivation, "brownouts"—a need to nap at any cost.

Toxicity: A constant feeling of being sick or unwell, hypothetically one of the results of the production and release by the protozoa of a substance which disorders the normal function of some organ or system. It may result in lack of concentration, confused memory, impaired motivation, nightmares, musculoskeletal pains, wide swings in blood sugar levels and menstrual irregularities.

In all cases, the severity of symptoms depends on a person's natural resistance, the amount of innoculum, secondary bacterial infections, and the host's nutritional status. It is interesting to note that these symptoms also appear in many of today's controversial diagnoses, such as Candidiasis, Epstein-Barr Virus and CMV. Frequently these diagnoses are made out of frustration. The practitioner does not have a clear clinical picture and can't get any positive procedural or lab results to be more specific.

The poor response of some of these patients may be due to a protozoal infection that has been missed or inadequately treated. I have successfully treated a significant number of patients with chronic candidiasis by controlling the protozoal infection. Restoring the integrity of the intestinal mucosa removes the unhealthy and fertile environment for yeast growth. I have also had success with patients with the "trash-basket diagnoses" of irritable bowel syndrome (IBS) and chronic fatigue syndrome (CFS).

These diagnoses inherently imply an emotional etiology when 15 percent, conservatively estimated, have a treatable protozoal infection. These patients' protracted unwellness is due in part to the lack of their practitioners' awareness of the prevalence of these diseases, and in part to their too easy acceptance of negative stool reports for ova and parasites.

Proper Diagnostic Use of the Rectal Swab Technique (RST)

The proper method of diagnosing these diseases is first getting a pertinent clinical history, with emphasis on date of onset of symptoms, in relation to the patient's travel or residential history. Lab reports are critical for a practitioner inexperienced in this field. Unfortunately, these reports are notoriously false negative for several reasons—the specimen is fecal matter which represents only the contents of the bowel lumen; the specimen is not fresh; and the technician is not adequately trained.

Before they closed in the 1980s due to New York's financial crisis, the public health tropical disease labs were very accurate. After that, several Manhattan labs specialized in parasitological diseases and did purge stool exams. Although these are much better specimens and a certain percent of false negatives are to be expected, I was dissatisfied, particularly in my own case, with repeated negative reports when clinically I knew I was infected.

By necessity I initiated the rectal swab technique (RST), which is basically a superficial biopsy, and discovered the protozoa myself in my own sample. The RST is far more accurate than casual stool exams and at least 25 percent more accurate and more practical than purged stool exams. Another benefit is the use of the anoscope, which allows examination of mucosal integrity. With an experienced technician immediately at hand, the results and treatment, if necessary, can be discussed in a single office visit.

Treatment

Success in treating these parasitic infections depends on a variety of factors, including length of time of infection, natural resistance, patient cooperation, repeated exposures, etc. My clinical impression is that the length of time needed to obtain a "satisfactory" result is related conceptually to the time the patient has been infected and gone untreated. In most cases I have treated, repeated courses are necessary just to establish control.

"Satisfactory" results are often the removal or reduction of severity of the symptoms, so that the patient is able to lead a life with acceptable bowel habits and normal energy. This does not mean that the parasites have been totally eliminated, which I have found is accomplished in only about 20 to 40 percent of the cases, an efficacy reflecting the length of an infestation before therapeutic intervention.

Medicines Available

I do not think one medicine is superior, but efficacy is dependent on consecutive ongoing courses of different protozides and combinations. The medication, dosage and length of a course of treatment must all be individualized to the patient's tolerance of the drugs and his or her lifestyle. The management of cases varies and frequently evokes a practitioner's creativity. Medicines for Amoebiasis are idoquinol, paramomycin-Humatin, and the tetracyclines.

Lilly recently ceased marketing the arsenical Carbarsonc, because they "didn't feel there was a need for an amoebicide." For Giardiasis there are quinacrine-Atabrine and furazolidone-Furozone. For both there is metronizadole-Flagyl. I do not feel it is essential for the successful treatment of the Protozoal Syndrome, but if tolerated it should be included as a single or repeated course in a therapeutic regimen.

My patients have taught me that the endpoint of therapy is not a negative lab report, but an improvement in or restoration of their quality of life. I have found that in a majority of improved cases, the lab reports may still be positive for protozoa, but the patient feels well. What appears to occur is that, with treatment, the protozoa are integrated into the several hundred other organisms alive in a natural flora of the intestinal tract. There is still a possibility that stress will bring a recurrence, but then therapy can be resumed, along with emphasis on rebuilding the immune system once again.

Counseling Patients on Prevention

Treatment should be accompanied by counseling against reinfection, including advice to avoid salads and uncooked dishes such as sushi or fresh fruit compotes when dining out, drinking only bottled beverages, and foregoing scatological sexual practices. People travelling abroad or in our national parks and wilderness areas should also boil or microfilter any non-bottled drinking water, or use several drops of an oxygenating liquid such as Acrox, which has been reported to kill the organisms through the addition of oxygen to the water, and also to take preventive medications.

Conclusions

Amoebiasis and Giardiasis are only recently being recognized as a forgotten cause of long-term illness in millions of Americans. The allopathic medical community has by undefinable social and scientific attitudes perfunctorily rejected these illnesses, and too frequently accepted false negative lab results as fact.

The wide variety of gastrointestinal symptoms, fatigue, and general toxicity can compromise a clinical picture and make these infections hard to diagnose.

The few drugs available to treat protozoal infections can have intolerable side effects and often do not eradicate the pathogens.

Millions are suffering from the symptoms of the Protozoal Syndrome and, even after medical evaluations, are unaware of the real cause of their problem—the protozoa. Once diagnosed and properly treated, most can be restored to health.

Reprinted by permission of *The Nutrition & Dietary Consultant*, March 1991.

A Brief Update of the Current Global Parasitic Epidemic

Geography and under-development are no longer the only criteria accounting for parasitic infestation. The most updated evaluations indicate that over 600 million people worldwide are infected with Amoebiasis, 300 million with Giardiasis, and over 100 million with Dientamoebiasis. A conservative estimate of the continental United States infection rate is 60 percent (30% Amoebiasis, 20% Giardiasis, and 10% Dientamoebiasis). Contributing factors are local water supplies, the third world influx into major cosmopolitan areas, and travel abroad.

If you have ever been ill while on a foreign vacation and suffered the symptoms of parasite infestation, including diarrhea, nausea, fatigue and other symptoms, there is a good possibility that *you may still have a parasite problem, even though the symptoms may have disappeared.*

A Perspective of Modern Anti-Pathogenic Therapeutic Modalities

Recently, due to an outbreak of a very malignant chloroquine-resistant malaria, the investigators of the World Health Organization have been instituting therapy with Artemesia Annua Vera, achieving surprising and dramatic results.

Because of these positive results, many authorities in the field are currently endeavoring to isolate the active agents responsible for this malaricidal effect. So far over 500 different chemical compounds have been isolated from this natural herb, many of them with antiparasitic activity.

Instituting a great deal of this research, Dr. Herman Bueno has achieved many scientific breakthroughs and discoveries. He has pioneered the use of Artemesia and other equally effective but less well-known herbs for a variety of modalities, which are discussed in the following pages.

Parasitic Disease Incidences Worldwide

from GEO Magazine, June 1984

Disease	Symptoms	People Infected	People with Symptoms	Deaths per Year
Roundworm	Intestinal obstruction	1,000,000,000	1,000,000	20,000
Hookworm	Anemia	900,000,000	1,500,000	50,000
Malaria	Fever, coma	800,000,000	150,000,000	1,200,000
Trichuriasis	Intestinal disease	500,000,000	10,000	Low
Amoebiasis	Dysentery	400,000,000	1,500,000	30,000
Filariasis	Elephantiasis	250,000,000	3,000,000	Low
Giardiasis	Diarrhea	200,000,000	500,000	Very Low
Bilharziasis	Liver/urinary fibrosis	200,000,000	20,000,000	750,000
Onchocerciasis	Blindness	30,000,000	500,000	35,000
Trypanosomiasis:				
South American	Heart disease	12,000,000	1,200,000	60,000
African	Sleeping sickness	1,000,000	10,000	5,000
Leishmanjasis	Sores, fever, anemia	12,000,000	12,000,000	5,000

Parasite Questionnaire

1. Have you ever developed diarrhea or abdominal distress while visiting a foreign country or another part of the U.S.? Yes ___ No ___

2. Is the consistency of your bowel movement changeable—sometimes hard and then soft for no apparent reason? Yes ___ No ___

3. Do you have unexplained periods of indigestion? Yes ___ No ___

4. Do you frequently feel bloated or gaseous for no apparent reason? Yes ___ No ___

5. Does your intestinal tract burn, cramp or feel irritable for no apparent reason? Yes ___ No ___

6. Do you have periods of fatigue for no apparent reason? Yes ___ No ___

7. Do you develop frequent colds, flu or other acute illnesses? Yes ___ No ___

8. Have you developed allergies to foods and environment in recent years? Yes ___ No ___

9. Do you have a recurring feeling of unwellness? Yes ___ No ___

10. Do you have a recurring candida overgrowth problem? Yes ___ No ___

If you answered yes to 5 or more of these questions, you may want to have your doctor order a laboratory test for parasites. *Even though the test may come back negative, there is still a strong possibility that parasites may be present.*

Laboratory Description of Common Parasites

Giardia lamblia: Giardia is a pathogenic lumen dwelling protozoa which parasitizes the upper intestinal tract. The trophozoite is the active parasitic form, but often only the cysts appear in the rectum. Giardia may cause gastrointestinal disturbances, food intolerances, fatigue, immunologic dysfunction and malabsorption. Treatment of giardiasis is recommended even in asymptomatic individuals because of the risk of activation and spread.

Entamoeba histolytica: This organism parasitizes the human large intestine and may cause bowel disturbances, food intolerance, fatigue and immunologic dysfunction. Pathogenicity depends upon the strain of amoeba. Migration of the organism to the liver and brain may occur concomitant with very heavy infestation of especially invasive strains.

Entamoeba hartmanni: Formerly called the "small race" of E. histolytica, the pathogenicity of this organism falls into a grey area of some dispute. As for histolytica, pathogenicity may relate to the specific strain.

Cryptosporidium: This is a minute coccidian parasite with worldwide distribution. It parasitizes the entire small and large intestine. In immunocompetent patients, symptomatic cryptosporidiosis generally produces a self-limited diarrhea and occasionally abdominal discomfort, anorexia, fever, nausea and weight loss. In immunodeficient patients, severe diarrhea and systemic symptoms are typical and the organism has been associated with malabsorption and hematogenous spread. The usual antiparasitic drugs are ineffective against cryptosporidiosis. In 1993, 430,000 people in Milwaukee fell ill from this protozoa. More than 125 died and many remain ill. This outbreak took place because the water district's usual method of filtration and chemicals used to kill bacteria and parasites does not effectively kill cryptosporidium. As of this date, none of the water districts across the U.S. have an effective method of eliminating this parasite from drinking water. For this reason you are urged not to drink tap water that is not properly filtered. An outbreak can happen anywhere.

Blastocystis hominis: The taxonomic status of this organism is unclear. Its pathogenicity appears to be low, although it has been implicated as a cause of chronic diarrhea in travellers. Blastocystis may not require treatment unless the infestation is very heavy and gastrointestinal or immunologic dysfunction is evident.

Endolimax nana: This is a common lumen dwelling protozoa which has generally been considered nonpathogenic. Reactive arthritis provoked by Endolimax infection has been reported, so that treatment is warranted in individuals with active inflammatory disorders.

Entamoeba coli: This is a common nonpathogenic protozoan. Its presence in the rectal swab indicates exposure to food or water contaminated with feces, but is not, in itself, an indication for treatment.

Iodamoeba butschli: This uncommon amoeba is generally nonpathogenic and treatment is usually not warranted.

Trichomonas hominis: The presence of this organism is indicative of direct fecal contamination, but there is no evidence it plays a pathogenic role in humans.

Dientamoeba fragilis: This organism may be pathogenic, causing bowel disturbances and immunologic dysfunction. Treatment of Dientamoeba fragilis is generally indicated.

Yeasts: Most yeasts found in the intestinal mucosa are described as dimorphic, in that they can exist in two states: the vegetative state usually referred to as hyphal, and the budding form where individual cells replicate by mitotic budding. The hyphal form is usually considered pathogenic, whereas the presence of a small number of budding yeasts is probably normal. Following is a glossary of frequently used terms:

Blastoconidium: A conidium formed by budding along a hypha, pseudohypha, or single cell, as in the yeasts.

Chlamydoconidium: A conidium that is thick walled and contains stored food. It may be located at the end of the hypha (terminally) or inserted along the hypha, singly or in chains.

Chlamydospore: A thick-walled vesicle formed by Candida albicans. It neither germinates nor produces conidia when mature.

Conidium (pl. conidia): Asexual propagule that forms on the side or end of the hypha or conidiophore. It may consist of one or more cells, and the size, shape, and arrangement in groups are generally characteristic of the organism.

Hypha (pl. hyphae): A tubular or threadlike structure of a fungus. Many together form a mycelium.

Mycelium (pl. mycelia): A mat or intertwined hyphae that constitutes the colony of a fungus.

Pseudohyphae: Chains of cells formed by budding that, when elongated, resemble true hyphae. They differ from true hyphae by being constricted at the septa, forming branches that begin with septation and having terminal cells smaller than the other cells.

Common Parasitic Diseases

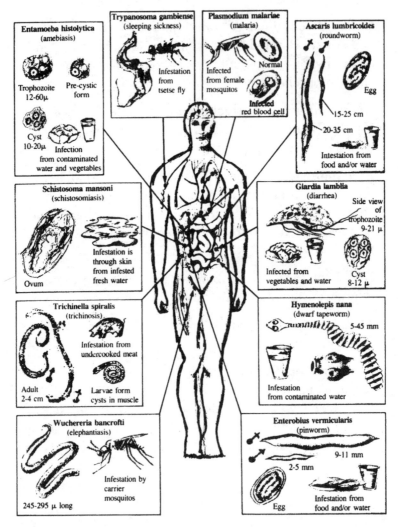

The above diagram illustrates ten common parasites, their source, and the areas of the body they are most likely to affect. Contaminated water is the most common breeding ground for parasites, and many water supplies in the U.S.A. are known to contain Giardia lamblia. Whenever possible, drink purified water. Avoid drinking river and stream water unless it is properly treated.

10

A New Generation of Herbal Parasite Fighters Has Arrived!

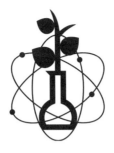

Presenting . . .
The Healing Within *Parasite Elimination Program*

The *Healing Within* Parasite Elimination Program consists of three groups of powerful herbal products and regular colon cleansings:

- **The Colon Complements:** Gozarte, Udarte, Neo-Pararte, Pasaloc, Padapco, K-Min, Black Walnut Tincture, Castor Oil Capsules, Intestinal Cleanser, and Latero Flora
- **Immune System Strengtheners:** Echinacea, Shitake Mushroom Capsules, and DDS Acidophilus
- **Post-Program Maintenance:** Intestinalis Herbal Cleanser
- **Colon Cleansings:** Colonic irrigation and enemas hasten expulsion of waste. Try to have a colonic once a week during the program to flush out parasites and other toxins. If colonics are not available in your area, give yourself a home enema twice a week.

The Colon Complements

All five herbal combinations—Gozarte, Udarte, Neo-Pararte, Pasaloc and Padapco—are the highest quality and most potent herbs available for parasite elimination. The herbs are organically grown in the tropical rain forests of Columbia without the use of pesticides or chemical fertilizers. These safe, effective and non-toxic therapeutic herbal agents have been produced after many years of research by Herman Bueno, M.D., a renowned parasitologist and member of the American Society of Tropical Medicine and Hygiene.

Some of the Organisms Affected by Gozarte, Udarte, Neo-Pararte, Pasaloc, and Padapco

Gozarte, Udarte, Neo-Pararte, Pasaloc, and Padapco have an extremely broad spectrum of activity. The following is a list of some affected organisms:

Entamoeba histolytica	Dientamoeba fragiles
Giardia lamblia	Causitive organisms for malaria
Blastocystis hominus	Schistosoma
Nematodes	Oxuilus vermicularis
Alcaligones faecalis	Enterobacter eloacae
Pseudomonas aeruginosa	Flavobacterium spp.
Micrococcus spp.	Alpha streptococci
Streptococcus pyogones	Chaetomium elatum
Salmonella typhosa	Bacillus subtillus
Brucella arbortus	Aspergillus niger
Pullularia pullulans	Staphylococcus aureus
Staphylococcus pyogenes	Staphylococcus saprophyticus
Staphylococcus faecalies	Bacillus subtilis
Bacillus mycoides	Cryptosporidium

Gram-Negative Bacteria

Proteus mirabilis	Proteus vulgaris
Escherichia coli	Salmonella anatum
Salmonella choleraesuis	Salmonella typhi
Salmonella paratyphi	Salmonella schorttmuelleri
Shigella dysenteriae	Pseudomonas aeruginosa

Ammonia Producers

Proteus miragilis	Proteus vulgaris
Brevibacterium ammoniagenes	

Facultative dermatophytes

Trichophyton gypseum	Trichophyton interdigital
Trichophyton rubrum	Epidermophyton floecosum
Candida albicans	

Fungi

Aspergillus niger	Aspergillus oryzae
Aspergillus terreus	Penicillium citrium
Penicillium funiculosum	Penicillium sp.
Penicillium rogueforti	Pullularia pullulans
Candida albicans	

• Gozarte

Gozarte is a natural herbal mixture of 500 mg. of Artemesia Annus Vera conjugated to 100 mg. of Gossypol. This combination provides an extremely potent broad spectrum antiparasitic agent. Gozarte is absorbed rapidly from the gastrointestinal tract into the bloodstream and is active locally and systemically within minutes after swallowing. It is a very effective agent and can be given concomitantly or independently with other herbs such as Neo-Pararte, Udarte and other parasite fighters. Gram for gram, Gozarte is 10 times more potent than Flagyl and Paramomcin and 1,000 times more potent than Diodoquin, with no side effects. It is a broad spectrum antiprotozoal agent specifically effective against Entamoeba histolytica, Giardia lamblia and Dientamoeba fragiles, malaria, tapeworms, fungicidal activity and Herpes II. Refer to Parasite Elimination Kits A1, B1 or C1, depending on your body weight.

In a chronic case of parasite infestation lasting more than 3 months, Neo-Pararte or Udarte should be taken in conjunction with Gozarte and the other parasite fighters for maximum results. Refer to Parasite Elimination Kits A3, B3 or C3, or A5, B5 or C5, depending on your body weight.

Adverse reactions are dose dependent and disappear upon discontinuation of the product. Herxheimer (die-off) reaction may occur with any effective parasitic elimination therapy.

There are no known side effects. Gozarte is not recommended for pregnant or lactating women.

Take Gozarte with food to avoid gastric upset. Reduce all anti-oxidant supplements to *no more* than the following daily dosages while taking Gozarte:

Vitamin A–25,000 units	Iron–Less than 100 mg.
Vitamin C–1000 mg.	Germanium–30 mg.
Vitamin E–400 I.U.	

Discontinue all other antioxidants while on this program. Antioxidants in high dosages reduce the potency of Gozarte, an Artemesia product, thus making it less effective. Avoid alcoholic and carbonated beverages while taking Gozarte.

• Neo-Pararte

Neo-Pararte is a natural herbal mixture of 400 mg. Artemesia Annua Vera conjugated to both 100 mg. DF-100 (an extract of grapefruit seed) and Lemoncillo 500 mg. This combination is an extremely effective and efficient broad spectrum anti-parasitic agent.

Neo-Pararte is absorbed rapidly from the gastrointestinal tract into the bloodstream, and is active both locally and systemically within one-half hour after taking. It is a very effective agent and can be used concomitantly with herbs such as Gozarte and other parasite fighters.

In a chronic case of parasite infestation lasting more than 3 months, Neo-Pararte should be taken in conjunction with Gozarte and the other *Healing Within* parasite fighters for maximum results. Refer to Parasite Elimination Kits A3, B3 or C3, depending on your body weight.

Adverse reactions are dose dependent and disappear upon discontinuation of the product. Herxheimer (die-off) reaction may occur with any effective parasitic elimination therapy. There are no known side effects. Neo-Pararte is not recommended for pregnant or lactating women.

Take Neo-Pararte with food to avoid gastric upset. Reduce all antioxidant supplements to *no more* than the following daily dosages while taking Neo-Pararte:

Vitamin A–25,000 units   Iron–Less than 100 mg.

Vitamin C–1000 mg.   Germanium–30 mg.

Vitamin E–400 I.U.

Discontinue all other antioxidants while on this program. Antioxidants in high dosages reduce the potency of Neo-Pararte, an Artemesia product, thus making it less effective. Avoid alcoholic and carbonated beverages while taking Neo-Pararte.

• *Udarte*

Udarte is a natural herbal mixture of Artemisia Annua (Vera) and AC Factor of plant source (Pringamoza). It is obtained from a Colombian variety of a uticaraceie plant. This combination provides an extremely potent broad spectrum antiparasitic as well as anticandida agent. The antichitin element, or AC Factor, destroys the cellular membrane of parasites and yeast with a catastrophic effect on those organisms.

Udarte is absorbed rapidly into the bloodstream and is active locally and systemically within minutes after swallowing. It is a very effective agent and should be taken concomitantly with Gozarte and the other *Healing Within* parasite fighters.

In a chronic case of parasite infestation and candida overgrowth lasting more than 3 months, Udarte should be taken in conjunction with Gozarte and the other *Healing Within* parasitic fighters for maximum results. Refer to Parasite Elimination Kits A5, B5 or C5, depending on your body weight.

Adverse reactions are dose dependent and disappear upon discontinuation of the product. Herxheimer (die-off) reaction may occur with an effective parasitic and candida elimination therapy. There are no known side effects. Udarte is not recommended for pregnant or lactating women.

Take Udarte with food to avoid gastric upset. Reduce all antioxidant supplements to *no more* than the following daily dosages while taking Udarte:

Vitamin A–25,000 units   Iron–Less than 100 mg.
Vitamin C–1000 mg.   Germanium–30 mg.
Vitamin E–400 I.U.

Discontinue all other antioxidants while on this program. Antioxidants in high dosages reduce the potency of Udarte, an Artemesia product, thus making it less effective. Avoid alcoholic and carbonated beverages while taking Udarte.

• *Pasaloc*

Pasaloc is a natural herbal mixture of E. Longitdia Colombianensis, Salvia Officinalis Colombianensis, and Malva Colombianensis (500 mg. per capsule). These herbs, grown in the rain forests of Colombia, are an extremely effective and efficient broad spectrum systemic antiparasitic combination. Pasaloc can be used concomitantly with other parasite-fighting herbs.

Note that Pasaloc does *not* contain the herb Artemesia Annua. Large dosages of oxygen-containing products such as Vitamins A, C, E, Iron, and Germanium can inhibit the strength and effectiveness of Artemesia-based products such as Gozarte, Udarte, and Neo-Pararte. Thus, if you wish to take large amounts of antioxidants and oxygen-containing products while on the Parasite Elimination Program, your choice should be Pasaloc, since it doesn't contain Artemesia Annua. Refer to Parasite Elimination Kits A2, B2, and C2, depending on your body weight.

In a chronic case of parasite infestation lasting more than 3 months, the herb Pasaloc should be taken in conjunction with Padapco and the other *Healing Within* parasite fighters for maximum results. Refer to Parasite Elimination Kits A4, B4 or C4, depending on your body weight.

Adverse reactions are dose dependent and disappear upon

discontinuation of the product. Herxheimer (die-off) reaction may occur with any effective parasitic elimination therapy. There are no known side effects to Pasaloc. Pasaloc is not recommended for pregnant or lactating women. Take Pasaloc with food to avoid gastric upset. Avoid alcoholic and carbonated beverages while taking this product.

• *Padapco*

Padapco is a natural herbal mixture of equal amounts of Daphentin A.D., Axantorryzia Colombianensis and Citrus Paradisi (500 mg. per capsule). These herbs, grown in the rain forests of Colombia, are an extremely effective and efficient broad spectrum systemic anti-parasitic combination. Padapco can be used concomitantly with other parasite-fighting herbs.

Note that Padapco does *not* contain the herb Artemesia Annua. Large dosages of oxygen-containing products such as Vitamins A, C, E, Iron, and Germanium can inhibit the strength and effectiveness of Artemesia-based products such as Gozarte, Udarte, and Neo-Pararte. Thus, if you wish to take large amounts of antioxidants and oxygen-containing products while on the Parasite Elimination Program, your choice should be Padapco, since it doesn't contain Artemesia Annua.

In a chronic case of parasite infestation lasting more than 3 months, the herb Padapco should be taken in conjunction with Pasaloc and the other *Healing Within* parasite fighters for maximum results. Refer to Parasite Elimination Kits A4, B4 or C4, depending on your body weight.

Adverse reactions are dose dependent and disappear upon discontinuation of the product. Herxheimer (die-off) reaction may occur with any effective parasitic elimination therapy. There are no known side effects to Padapco. Padapco is not recommended for pregnant or lactating women. Take Padapco with food to avoid gastric upset. Avoid alcoholic and carbonated beverages while taking this product.

Recommendations

See pages 238-241 for an itemization of all the products in the *Healing Within* Parasite Elimination Kits. A price list for these kits, as well as individual items, begins on page 291.

If you have been affected by parasites for less than 3 months, use Kits A1, B1 or C1 (depending on your body weight), all of which contain Gozarte. However, you must reduce antioxidant supplements such as Vitamins A, C, E, Iron, and Germanium. If you wish to continue taking large dosages of these supplements, use Kits A2, B2 or C2 (depending on your body weight), all of which contain Pasaloc instead of Gozarte. Antioxidant supplements will not interfere with the effectiveness of Pasaloc.

If you have had a parasite problem for *more* than 3 months, it would be considered a chronic condition. In this case, use Kits A3, B3 or C3 (depending on your body weight), all of which contain Gozarte and Neo-Pararte. If you have parasites as well as candida (or a history of candida problems), use Kits A5, B5 or C5 (depending on your body weight). However, you must reduce antioxidant supplements such as Vitamins A, C, E, Iron, and Germanium. If you wish to continue taking large dosages of these supplements, use Kits A4, B4 or C4 (depending on your body weight), all of which contain Pasaloc and Padapco. Antioxidant supplements will not interfere with the effectiveness of Pasaloc and Padapco.

Gozarte, Udarte, Neo-Pararte, Pasaloc, and Padapco work very efficiently; so efficiently, in fact, that they may cause a die-off reaction. Having a colonic irrigation or suspending the program for a day or two will probably relieve the symptoms. You can effectively deal with nausea from die-off reactions by taking the natural herb Stinging Nettles (Urtica Dioica).

• K-Min

K-Min is a combination product of elements gathered above the earth and mined from the earth. K-Min will, by ionization, take worms apart; rarely will parasites pass out of the body whole. K-Min is a very effective compound in removing parasites from the intestinal tract. When the intestinal tract is free of parasites, yeast infection will usually clear up. The combination of K-Min and Black Walnut Tincture is effective against fungi, skin infections (due to microscopic parasites), ringworms, and larvae from the large intestine.

• Black Walnut Tincture

Black Walnut Tincture is an herbal fluid that fights parasites throughout the body. When tension is present in the intestinal tract, Black Walnut Tincture is a tremendously soothing healant and is an excellent source of manganese. The elements in Black Walnut Tincture are unsurpassed for helping to strengthen ligaments, tendons and muscles. *Indian Herbology of North America* states that Black Walnut Tincture assists in the healing of acne, burning in the anus, pain over the eyes, gas, headaches, herpes, scurvy, and pain in the spleen, as well as syphilis, ulcers, rickets, and TB.

• Castor Oil Capsules

Castor oil, when encapsulated and frozen, will pass through the stomach and small intestine before dissolving. Freezing castor oil capsules before ingesting totally eliminates the traditional cramping associated with this product, because the capsules dissolve in the ileum, the last three-fifths of the small intestine. Here the digestive tract hydrolizes this oil into recinoleic acid, which is harmless to humans but deadly to parasites.

The ileum connects to the cecum by way of the ileocecal valve. The majority of parasites of all kinds will nest in the cecum area (the lower end of the ascending colon where the large bowel begins). This area is warm and moist, providing a plentiful source of fresh food for these poisonous invaders.

Castor oil not only suffocates parasites, but is nature's penetrating oil for colon plaque. When the Castor Oil Capsule is *frozen* it does not act as a laxative. Castor oil is odorless and will not "burp" back.

• Healing Within *Intestinal Cleanser*

Healing Within Intestinal Cleanser pulls mucous, detoxifies, heals, acts as a diuretic, activates flushing of the liver and production of bile, and improves intestinal peristalsis. *Healing Within* Intestinal Cleanser contains the following ingredients:

Bentonite

Bentonite, a totally natural product of Mother Earth, is microscopic and carries a large and varied mineral content. This particular strain of bentonite is unequaled in controlling conditions of diarrhea where virus infections, food allergies, spastic colitis, and food poisoning exist. "Bentonite carries a strong negative electron and picks up 12 times its weight in positively charged toxic material from the colon wall for expulsion. The action of bentonite is purely physical and not chemical. Bentonite is used as a treatment of intestinal fermentation (gas), putrefaction, and harmful bacteria as well as parasites." (Medical Annuals of Washington, D.C., Vol. 20(6), June, 1961, The Value of Bentonite.)

Wheat Grass

Dr. Birscher, research scientist, calls wheat grass chlorophyll "concentrated Sun Power." Wheat grass also carries a negative electron and picks up eight times its weight in positively charged toxic material from the intestinal walls for expulsion. Wheat grass is known to increase the function of the heart, vascular system, intestines, uterus, and lungs. The wheat grass chlorophyll "raises the basic nitrogen exchange and is, therefore, a tonic without comparison." The gentle roughage of wheat grass releases clinging debris from intricate crevices of the bowel.

Apple Fiber

Chemical-free apples make up apple fiber, which is loaded

with vitamins, minerals, proteins, and life-saving pectin and lipids. Apple fiber gently "brushes" and cleanses the intestinal wall, while the apple seeds provide nitrilosides.

Citrus Pectin and Plantago Avato

These products capture putrefactive bacteria for expulsion. The jelling effect of pectin and plantago avato make them especially advantageous in this formula. The two are invaluable in forming a gentle colloidal mass for capturing and holding in suspension the impacted toxic material pulled from the walls of the colon. Citrus pectin is known for releasing heavy metals, such as mercury and lead, from the cells for expulsion. Citrus pectin is reported to help counteract the effects of radiation, cut cholesterol in blood, and reduce risk of heart attacks.

Herbs

Nature's natural medicines are part of the plan for man's survival. *Healing Within* Intestinal Cleanser contains gentian, golden seal, buckthorn, rhubarb root, cascara sagrada, and aloe vera, all well calculated and delicately balanced in proportions essential for the success of the cleanser and detoxifier.

Lactobacillus Acidophilus

Acidophilus is essential for balancing body chemistry. The purpose of acidophilus in this formula is to reinforce the production of healthy bacteria in the colon. Where there is too little acidophilus, gas forms, stools become putrid, and the normal production of Vitamin K is destroyed. When Vitamin K is destroyed, internal hemorrhaging can occur. When folic acid becomes deficient, the body cannot manufacture enough maintenance B-complex to stabilize the nerves, and thus energy levels diminish and halitosis tells the sordid story.

• *Latero Flora*

Latero Flora is extremely effective for individuals with gastrointestinal disturbances, food allergies, and candidiasis hypersensitivity syndrome. Latero Flora normalizes the flora in the human digestive tract, aids in digestion and toxin elimination, and discourages the growth of yeast, fungi and other pathogenic microorganisms. Latero Flora restores the original, desirable bacterial balance to human intestines, thus improving many immuno-suppressed conditions.

Luc DeSchepper, M.D., Ph.D., C.A., studied the "before and after" symptoms of 1,500 patients suffering from chronic fatigue, along with a wide variety of immuno-suppressive symptoms. Dr. DeSchepper made his report in the *Townsend Letter for Doctors:* "Latero Flora has shown significant effectiveness in improving and in many cases eliminating gastrointestinal symptoms and food sensitivities, while enhancing the patient's digestive capacities . . . I am convinced that Latero Flora will play a very important role in fighting the scourge of this century—the suppression of the immune system."

Immune System Strengtheners

The immune system is one of the most complex systems of the human body. Until recently, researchers, scientists and physicians have had little understanding of the structure and function of this system. The basic components are the lymphatic system, white blood cells and their specialized groups, and the antibody mechanisms of the specialized organs.

Scientists are gaining a better understanding of the immune system and what it takes to biochemically aid and support its function. Many of these biochemical components are found in valuable herbs and botanical extracts which contain nutrients that are essential in nourishing the glands that regulate the function and detoxification of the immune system.

• Echinacea

One of the most outstanding herbs for strengthening the immune system is Echinacea angustifolia. Studies in Europe and America have shown that the chemical compounds in Echinacea have anti-inflammatory action while stimulating the healing of wounds. Echinacea has also been shown to stimulate white blood cells and lymphocytes, making it effective against viral and bacterial infections. Echinacea is effective internally or externally, and has no side effects. Parasite Elimination Kits contain a 6-week supply.

• Shitake Mushroom Capsules

For centuries in China and Japan, shitake mushrooms have been recognized as a nutritious food and highly esteemed as a home remedy for many ailments. Shitake Mushroom Capsules exhibit a wide spectrum of beneficial effects on the immune system, and are anti-viral, anti-fungal, anti-inflammatory as well as anti-protozoal. They have been known to lower cholesterol and are an excellent candida fighter. Echinacea and Shitake will help to strengthen the immune system and reduce fatigue associated with parasitic problems. *Healing Within* Parasite Elimination Kits contain a 6-week supply.

• Acidophilus

Taking an Acidophilus culture during this 60-day program is highly recommended, as it will restore the good bacteria that have been destroyed by antibiotics and parasitic infestation. DDS Acidophilus is capable of producing B vitamins and reducing cholesterol. It helps with food digestion, especially dairy products, and is a natural antibiotic. DDS Acidophilus has been found to help inhibit the following organisms as well as retard the growth of *Candida albicans* (yeast infections).

Bacillus subtilis	Bacillus cereus
Bacillus stearothermophilus	Streptococcus faecalis var. liquifaciens
Streptococcus lactis	Lactobacillus lactis
Lactobacillus casei	Lactobacillus plantarum
Lactobacillus leichmannii	Sarcina lutea
Serratia marcescens	Proteus vulgaris
Escherichia coli	Salmonella typhosa

Salmonella schottmuelleri   Shigella dysenteriae
Shigella paradysenteriae   Pseudomonas fluorescens
Pseudomonas aeruginosa   Staphylococcus aureus
Klebsiella pneumoniae   Vibrio comma

Post-Program Maintenance

• *Intestinalis Herbal Cleanser*

Intestinalis is an excellent combination of 22 herbs to help maintain and protect the intestinal tract from reinfestation after you have completed the *Healing Within* 60-Day Parasite Elimination Program. Intestinalis is both an anti-parasitic and anti-candida agent, as well as a soothing tonic for the intestinal tract.

Letters from Satisfied Clients

May 28, 1991

Dear Stan:

I'm sorry to have taken so long to let you know about the effects of your parasite program. I wanted to observe myself for awhile in order to figure out where my various symptoms were coming from. What I learned was very interesting.

First of all, your program was very effective for getting my eliminations back to normal. For the first time in many years I am having regular bowel movements of a sort that I have not seen since I was a young adult, without any help from intestinal cleansers. Second, I no longer experience those very unpleasant feelings of internal congestion which seemed like some kind of chronic infection. In addition, the chest infection that plagued me for about one and a half years is gone.

These days I am feeling very well (although I have not yet regained all the weight I lost) because I am careful about what I eat. I want to tell you again how deeply grateful I am to you for making your products available to those of us who become ill and would otherwise have nowhere to turn for help because there is so little understanding of these problems within the medical profession. May all your ways prosper!

Yours sincerely,
Cora Scott

Dear Mr. Weinberger:

I'm pleased to tell you that I highly endorse both your Parasite and Candida eradication programs. Prior to treatment at Colon Health Center, I had both conditions at the same time. My health was so severely affected I could not be employed, not even part-time. The nausea, pain, dizziness, mental disorientation and respiratory distress transformed me into a socially isolated semi-invalid who left the house only twice a week when absolutely necessary to go to the bank or grocery store. And sometimes I had to delegate even those few chores to sympathetic friends, I was that weak! And I looked as terrible as I felt, as I also had a lot of insomnia.

After four years of illness, your programs did an excellent job of turning my situation around and bringing back normal body functioning. Since my case was extreme and stubborn, other programs failed me. Yours did not. Your approach towards eradicating these incapacitating health scourges is the most intensive I've used. Congratulations!

Sincerely,
Nell Roche
Santa Rosa, CA

June 15, 1991

Dear Mr. Weinberger:
I wanted to write to let you know how much I appreciate your efforts. For more than two years I was going to doctors, acupuncturists, homeopaths and herbalists in hopes of finding relief from my illness. Some of the treatments, in particular the acupuncture, seemed to help relieve my symptoms, but none were capable of providing more than temporary relief.

Diagnosed two years ago by my doctor as "having had" the Epstein-Barr virus, he indicated that it wasn't even possible to tell if the virus was still affecting me. Even it if was, he said, there was no treatment.

I am now certain, after your treatment, that while Epstein-Barr may not have been my immediate problem, it likely was the thing that allowed a parasitic infection to get a foothold in my system. The result: insomnia, hypoglycemic-type symptoms, weight loss, diarrhea, fatigue and nervousness.

I found the health center physicians almost totally ignorant about parasitic infections, and even incapable of diagnosing them properly. I tried your Parasite Elimination Program because I suspected that parasites might be the cause, but in all honesty I wasn't totally convinced. And, in the middle of the treatment, when my doubts surfaced, I was grateful for your reassurance during our phone conversations. The eventual results justify your assurance.

The change has been dramatic. I'm back to pursuing my avocation—photography—and I'm able to run errands without worrying about having an "attack" while out. In short, only two weeks after finishing the treatment, I have begun to feel "normal" for the first time in years. It's so great to see the light again. Hooray!

Many thanks,
Gay Marshall

November 13, 1992

Dear Stanley,
Eight years ago, at age 40, I retired as a Senior Army Officer, after twenty-two years of service. During the transition years the state of my health became the focus of my life. As I became a vegetarian, yogi and tantra yogi, I detoxified, colon cleansed and was therapied. I was Rolf'd, Heller'd, and Trager'd. Whatever was new and

237

hot was next. I was hooked. "Hello, my name is John, and I'm a healing addict."

So it was, several years later, that I arrived at your door with my chin on my chest and deeply exhausted. The great reserve of youthful vibrance and genetic strength that had seen me through the trials of my life was depleted. I was in breakdown.

The information that you shared enabled me to begin to recall the jungles and countrysides to which, as a special forces soldier, I had been sent; and the reactions of my body, to the foods and liquids offered to me, made sense. Finally I was clear. I still had parasites! The previous treatments had been ineffective; and my immune system was seriously inhibited. Thankfully my genetic predisposition for health supported me beyond the military. The thought of being in breakdown, and at the mercy of the Army Medical Corps is too horrific to ponder.

I have completed the Parasite Elimination Program and although my immune system is just beginning to heal, the changes are dramatic. I require less food and sleep for the same lifestyle. The bloating that I once experienced is gone. And, my body is more fit and toned.

Lastly, it was you, Stanley, the person and storehouse of knowledge, that made my choice to do the program an easy one. I sincerely appreciate your being there with me in those moments that were most challenging. Thanks for your support and love.

Warm regards,

John Freedom
Corte Madera, CA

December 18, 1992

Dear Stan:

I just wanted you to know how much I appreciate the help you have given me with my health. It is now about 4 months since I completed the parasite cleanse and I am steadily doing better.

I'm continuing to take the Dioxychlor, but am not really sure that I have a candida problem any more. After years of a major candida problem, it finally seems to be disappearing. I figure I'll stop taking the Dioxychlor on a gradual basis and see what happens.

I continue to gain in energy and well-being. For the last seven years I have had to go weekly to the chiropractor to stay in adjustment and keep away migraine headaches. Since completing the parasite cleanse and about 2 months into the Dioxychlor program, I was able to stop going to the chiropractor regularly and have only gone once in the last 3 months. There have been days I have felt totally healthy and then I get very excited because I get the idea of what it would be like to have no body problems at all. It seems clear that I am moving toward that and to an end to the distractions that the body has been these last 10 years.

Best wishes for the coming year,

Alexandra Hopkins
North Hollywood, CA

September 14, 1991

In 1991, I found myself depleted, fatigued, and plagued with digestive problems, chronic bloating, gas, and you name it. After trying several different therapies and approaches, Stanley Weinberger finally nailed it: parasites.

"Parasites!" I said, "But..." Stanley then explained it all to me.

"How can you possibly get rid of Candida, Epstein-Barr, the gas and bloating and digestive problems if you don't address your condition on the ground level?" he said. "The invasion of the parasites has lowered your immune system, creating the environment for the other conditions to enter into your weakened system. Then one thing led to another. You have to get rid of the parasites first, and then the other conditions will either disappear, improve, or at least you will be able to address them effectively."

I was so grateful to finally get the answers I had been searching for, as nobody had been able to explain my condition accurately to me. I immediately began Stanley's 60-Day Parasite Elimination Program.

There were days when I felt awful, and other days when I began to see the light at the end of the tunnel and felt my energy and enthusiasm returning. Whenever I felt really bad and clogged up, I would take a colonic and always felt relieved. And there were moments when I resisted the program. But with a call to Stanley and a few encouraging words from my coach, my doubts and fears vanished and I started up again.

I finished the program, and I'm now basically back to normal. Most of my conditions have either disappeared or diminished. Those that remain I can now deal with in a stronger, more cleaned-out state.

Stanley really knows what he is doing, and has the most up-to-date information on the best supplements and herbs to take. He is totally dedicated to healing and help-ing people all over the country, is impeccable in his prac-tice, and can be trusted to accurately pinpoint the area of concern. He's the best.

Constance Demby
San Anselmo, CA

Healing Within *Parasite Elimination Kits*

Parasite Elimination Kit Recommendations

Kit	Body Weight
A	Less than 100 lbs.
B	100-175 lbs.
C	More than 175 lbs.

If you have had parasites LESS than 3 months:

Kit A1, B1 or C1 with Gozarte	Reduce antioxidants to the amounts in the last chart below*
OR	
Kit A2, B2 or C2 with Pasaloc	Reduction of antioxidants is not required with these products

If you have had parasites MORE than 3 months:

Kit A3, B3 or C3 with Gozarte and Neo-Pararte	Reduce antioxidants to the amounts in the last chart below*
OR	
Kit A4, B4 or C4 with Pasaloc and Padapco	Reduction of antioxidants is not required with these products

If you have parasites *and* candida:

Kit A5, B5 or C5 with Gozarte and Udarte	Reduce antioxidants to the amounts in the last chart below*

* Reduce anti-oxidants to *no more* than the following amounts daily:

Vitamin A	25,000 units
Vitamin C	1000 mg.
Vitamin E	400 I.U.
Iron	Less than 100 mg.
Germanium	30 mg.
All other antioxidants	Discontinue while on program

60-Day Parasite Elimination Program Kits
— For body weight under 100 lbs. —

KIT A1 — Complete 60-Day Kit   19 Bottles Total — $ 529.00

1 Black Walnut Tincture (4 ounces each bottle)
2 Castor Oil (180 capsules each bottle)
2 DDS Acidophilus (100 capsules each bottle)
2 Echinacea (90 capsules each bottle)
3 Gozarte (60 capsules each bottle)

2 *Healing Within* Intestinal Cleanser
   (250 capsules each bottle)
1 Intestinalis Herbal Cleanser (60 tblts. each bottle)
2 K-Min (180 capsules each bottle)
2 Latero Flora (60 capsules each bottle)
2 Shitake Mushrooms (90 capsules each bottle)

KIT A2 — Complete 60-Day Kit   19 Bottles Total — $ 529.00

1 Black Walnut Tincture (4 ounces each bottle)
2 Castor Oil (180 capsules each bottle)
2 DDS Acidophilus (100 capsules each bottle)
2 Echinacea (90 capsules each bottle)
2 *Healing Within* Intestinal Cleanser
   (250 capsules each bottle)

1 Intestinalis Herbal Cleanser (60 tblts. each bottle)
2 K-Min (180 capsules each bottle)
2 Latero Flora (60 capsules each bottle)
3 Pasaloc (60 capsules each bottle)
2 Shitake Mushrooms (90 capsules each bottle)

KIT A3 — Complete 60-Day Kit   22 Bottles Total — $ 757.00

1 Black Walnut Tincture (4 ounces each bottle)
2 Castor Oil (180 capsules each bottle)
2 DDS Acidophilus (100 capsules each bottle)
2 Echinacea (90 capsules each bottle)
3 Gozarte (60 capsules each bottle)
2 *Healing Within* Intestinal Cleanser
   (250 capsules each bottle)

1 Intestinalis Herbal Cleanser (60 tblts. each bottle)
2 K-Min (180 capsules each bottle)
2 Latero Flora (60 capsules each bottle)
3 Neo-Pararte (60 capsules each bottle)
2 Shitake Mushrooms (90 capsules each bottle)

KIT A4 — Complete 60-Day Kit   22 Bottles Total — $ 757.00

1 Black Walnut Tincture (4 ounces each bottle)
2 Castor Oil (180 capsules each bottle)
2 DDS Acidophilus (100 capsules each bottle)
2 Echinacea (90 capsules each bottle)
2 *Healing Within* Intestinal Cleanser
   (250 capsules each bottle)

1 Intestinalis Herbal Cleanser (60 tblts. each bottle)
2 K-Min (180 capsules each bottle)
2 Latero Flora (60 capsules each bottle)
3 Padapco (60 capsules each bottle)
3 Pasaloc (60 capsules each bottle)
2 Shitake Mushrooms (90 capsules each bottle)

KIT A5 — Complete 60-Day Kit   22 Bottles Total — $ 757.00

1 Black Walnut Tincture (4 ounces each bottle)
2 Castor Oil (180 capsules each bottle)
2 DDS Acidophilus (100 capsules each bottle)
2 Echinacea (90 capsules each bottle)
3 Gozarte (60 capsules each bottle)
2 *Healing Within* Intestinal Cleanser
   (250 capsules each bottle)

1 Intestinalis Herbal Cleanser (60 tblts. each bottle)
2 K-Min (180 capsules each bottle)
2 Latero Flora (60 capsules each bottle)
2 Shitake Mushrooms (90 capsules each bottle)
3 Udarte (60 capsules each bottle)

**Detailed instructions for taking the products will be enclosed in your
Parasite Elimination Program Kit. See Order Form on page 291.**

60-Day Parasite Elimination Program Kits
— For body weight 100-175 lbs. —

KIT B1 — Complete 60-Day Kit   20 Bottles Total — $ 542.00

1 Black Walnut Tincture (4 ounces each bottle)
3 Castor Oil (180 capsules each bottle)
2 DDS Acidophilus (100 capsules each bottle)
2 Echinacea (90 capsules each bottle)
3 Gozarte (60 capsules each bottle)

2 *Healing Within* Intestinal Cleanser
   (250 capsules each bottle)
1 Intestinalis Herbal Cleanser (60 tblts. each bottle)
2 K-Min (180 capsules each bottle)
2 Latero Flora (60 capsules each bottle)
2 Shitake Mushrooms (90 capsules each bottle)

KIT B2 — Complete 60-Day Kit   20 Bottles Total — $ 542.00

1 Black Walnut Tincture (4 ounces each bottle)
3 Castor Oil (180 capsules each bottle)
2 DDS Acidophilus (100 capsules each bottle)
2 Echinacea (90 capsules each bottle)
2 *Healing Within* Intestinal Cleanser
   (250 capsules each bottle)

1 Intestinalis Herbal Cleanser (60 tblts. each bottle)
2 K-Min (180 capsules each bottle)
2 Latero Flora (60 capsules each bottle)
3 Pasaloc (60 capsules each bottle)
2 Shitake Mushrooms (90 capsules each bottle)

KIT B3 — Complete 60-Day Kit   23 Bottles Total — $ 770.00

1 Black Walnut Tincture (4 ounces each bottle)
3 Castor Oil (180 capsules each bottle)
2 DDS Acidophilus (100 capsules each bottle)
2 Echinacea (90 capsules each bottle)
3 Gozarte (60 capsules each bottle)
2 *Healing Within* Intestinal Cleanser
   (250 capsules each bottle)

1 Intestinalis Herbal Cleanser (60 tblts. each bottle)
2 K-Min (180 capsules each bottle)
2 Latero Flora (60 capsules each bottle)
3 Neo-Pararte (60 capsules each bottle)
2 Shitake Mushrooms (90 capsules each bottle)

KIT B4 — Complete 60-Day Kit   23 Bottles Total — $ 770.00

1 Black Walnut Tincture (4 ounces each bottle)
3 Castor Oil (180 capsules each bottle)
2 DDS Acidophilus (100 capsules each bottle)
2 Echinacea (90 capsules each bottle)
2 *Healing Within* Intestinal Cleanser
   (250 capsules each bottle)

1 Intestinalis Herbal Cleanser (60 tblts. each bottle)
2 K-Min (180 capsules each bottle)
2 Latero Flora (60 capsules each bottle)
3 Padapco (60 capsules each bottle)
3 Pasaloc (60 capsules each bottle)
2 Shitake Mushrooms (90 capsules each bottle)

KIT B5 — Complete 60-Day Kit   23 Bottles Total — $ 770.00

1 Black Walnut Tincture (4 ounces each bottle)
3 Castor Oil (180 capsules each bottle)
2 DDS Acidophilus (100 capsules each bottle)
2 Echinacea (90 capsules each bottle)
3 Gozarte (60 capsules each bottle)
2 *Healing Within* Intestinal Cleanser
   (250 capsules each bottle)

1 Intestinalis Herbal Cleanser (60 tblts. each bottle)
2 K-Min (180 capsules each bottle)
2 Latero Flora (60 capsules each bottle)
2 Shitake Mushrooms (90 capsules each bottle)
3 Udarte (60 capsules each bottle)

**Detailed instructions for taking the products will be enclosed in your
Parasite Elimination Program Kit. See Order Form on page 291.**

60-Day Parasite Elimination Program Kits
— For body weight over 175 lbs. —

KIT C1 — Complete 60-Day Kit   22 Bottles Total — $ 575.00

1 Black Walnut Tincture (4 ounces each bottle)
4 Castor Oil (180 capsules each bottle)
2 DDS Acidophilus (100 capsules each bottle)
2 Echinacea (90 capsules each bottle)
3 Gozarte (60 capsules each bottle)

3 *Healing Within* Intestinal Cleanser
  (250 capsules each bottle)
1 Intestinalis Herbal Cleanser (60 tblts. each bottle)
2 K-Min (180 capsules each bottle)
2 Latero Flora (60 capsules each bottle)
2 Shitake Mushrooms (90 capsules each bottle)

KIT C2 — Complete 60-Day Kit   22 Bottles Total — $ 575.00

1 Black Walnut Tincture (4 ounces each bottle)
4 Castor Oil (180 capsules each bottle)
2 DDS Acidophilus (100 capsules each bottle)
2 Echinacea (90 capsules each bottle)
3 *Healing Within* Intestinal Cleanser
  (250 capsules each bottle)

1 Intestinalis Herbal Cleanser (60 tblts. each bottle)
2 K-Min (180 capsules each bottle)
2 Latero Flora (60 capsules each bottle)
3 Pasaloc (60 capsules each bottle)
2 Shitake Mushrooms (90 capsules each bottle)

KIT C3 — Complete 60-Day Kit   25 Bottles Total — $ 803.00

1 Black Walnut Tincture (4 ounces each bottle)
4 Castor Oil (180 capsules each bottle)
2 DDS Acidophilus (100 capsules each bottle)
2 Echinacea (90 capsules each bottle)
3 Gozarte (60 capsules each bottle)
3 *Healing Within* Intestinal Cleanser
  (250 capsules each bottle)

1 Intestinalis Herbal Cleanser (60 tblts. each bottle)
2 K-Min (180 capsules each bottle)
2 Latero Flora (60 capsules each bottle)
3 Neo-Pararte (60 capsules each bottle)
2 Shitake Mushrooms (90 capsules each bottle)

KIT C4 — Complete 60-Day Kit   25 Bottles Total — $ 803.00

1 Black Walnut Tincture (4 ounces each bottle)
4 Castor Oil (180 capsules each bottle)
2 DDS Acidophilus (100 capsules each bottle)
2 Echinacea (90 capsules each bottle)
3 *Healing Within* Intestinal Cleanser
  (250 capsules each bottle)

1 Intestinalis Herbal Cleanser (60 tblts. each bottle)
2 K-Min (180 capsules each bottle)
2 Latero Flora (60 capsules each bottle)
3 Padapco (60 capsules each bottle)
3 Pasaloc (60 capsules each bottle)
2 Shitake Mushrooms (90 capsules each bottle)

KIT C5 — Complete 60-Day Kit   25 Bottles Total — $ 803.00

1 Black Walnut Tincture (4 ounces each bottle)
4 Castor Oil (180 capsules each bottle)
2 DDS Acidophilus (100 capsules each bottle)
2 Echinacea (90 capsules each bottle)
3 Gozarte (60 capsules each bottle)
3 *Healing Within* Intestinal Cleanser
  (250 capsules each bottle)

1 Intestinalis Herbal Cleanser (60 tblts. each bottle)
2 K-Min (180 capsules each bottle)
2 Latero Flora (60 capsules each bottle)
2 Shitake Mushrooms (90 capsules each bottle)
3 Udarte (60 capsules each bottle)

**Detailed instructions for taking the products will be enclosed in your
Parasite Elimination Program Kit. See Order Form on page 291.**

11

Metabolic Typing: The Commonsense Guide to Proper Nutrition

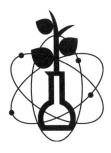

Metabolic Typing: The Commonsense Guide to Proper Nutrition

by William L. Wolcott

Many people have asked, "What do I need to do to achieve optimum health?" A large number of health-conscious individuals, failing to find proper guidance in the marketplace, discover for themselves that even by eating the very best organic foods and taking all the finest nutritional supplements money can buy, they still do not feel completely well. Moreover, what seems to work for some people, making them feel better or improving their adverse symptoms, in others has little or no effect, and in still others, actually appears to *worsen their health situation!*

If you (or anyone else for that matter) do not already know the answer to that question, finding out can prove to be an overwhelming undertaking. Little help of any real value can be gained from traditional medicine whose focus is on treating disease rather than on building health. A typical response from the average physician, when asked the above question, is to advise you to merely eat a well-balanced diet. But when you ask the next logical question, "What is a well-balanced diet for me?" you probably receive little, if any, meaningful information at all.

Creating Clarity from Confusion

Take heart, for there does appear to be a solution to all of this! Although we don't claim to have all the answers, HEALTHEXCEL has made an exciting and promising break-through by providing a framework for understanding what appears to be a hopeless morass of confusing and conflicting information about which foods to eat and which supplements to take in order to be healthy.

HEALTHEXCEL is an organization dedicated to the acceleration of the unfoldment of human potential through the creation of excellence in health. The basis for this unfoldment is a provocative, health-building program that is structured in an individualized approach to nutrition known as the HEALTHEXCEL System of Metabolic Typing.

You have probably heard it said, "You are what you eat." However, a much more accurate expression would be, "You are what you metabolize." Metabolism is the conversion of nutrients to energy, and the best way to know your unique nutritional needs is through an integrated approach of experimentation, observation, and the science of metabolic typing.

Metabolic typing is a highly complex procedure that requires the use of computer technology to analyze an enormous amount of personal data concerning each person's unique metabolic characteristics in order to determine individual nutritional requirements.

The concept of unique individual requirements for nutrition is certainly not an original idea brought forth by HEALTHEXCEL, nor even is the term "metabolic typing." The ancient Greek physicians, such as Hippocrates, recognized in their writings the validity of addressing the needs of the whole person, rather than just the symptoms of disease. To para-phrase their thinking on the subject, they recognized that different people had different kinds of maladies and that one man's food was another man's poison. Similar concepts can also be found in the ancient healing arts in the Far East, such as the yin and yang of Chinese medicine, and the correlation of the five elements to individual classifications in the Ayurvedic medicine of India.

Modern, progressive-minded researchers have revived this notion of health being dependent on our ability to obtain all the nutrients for which we have a genetic requirement. Dr. Roger Williams, the noted biochemist from the University of Texas, expounded his genetotrophic principle in which he showed that our individual characteristics, which are an expression of our uniqueness, are based in our genes and that these genetically inherited differences extend to even the level of the individual cell in determining the rate of individual cellular activity.

According to Dr. Williams, *all people are genetically predisposed to specific biochemical needs, which if not met, lead to degenerative disease.* This he termed a person's biochemical individuality. He believes that all degenerative disease, including cancer, is caused by such "cellular malnutrition."

Dr. Williams advocates the need ". . . to develop techniques for identifying the inherited pattern of susceptibilities and resistances that is unique to each individual. This metabolic profile represents a necessary precondition for making rational programs of nutrition, tailored to fit each individual's special requirements."

Other independent metabolic and nutritional researchers concurrently developed just such metabolic typing systems for the determination of individual nutritional requirements. Many researchers, such as Dr. Francis Pottenger and Dr. R. O. Muller, worked with individual classification through the autonomic nervous system. Dr. William Donald Kelley coined the term "metabolic typing" and was the first to utilize computer technology to analyze nutritional needs based on the autonomic nervous system. Dr. George Watson's research, and later that of Dr. Paul Eck, centered around the oxidation rate, the rate at which nutrients are burned for energy in the cells, as the basis for the determination of individual nutritional needs. Other researchers, such as Dr. Henry Bieler, Dr. Melvin Page, and Dr. Elliot Abravanel, developed means of classification through analysis of the endocrine system.

It has become quite clear that the acquisition of good health is dependent on good nutrition. It has also become quite clear that what is right for one person, as the ancient Greeks knew, is not necessarily correct for someone else. What constitutes good nutrition for the Eskimo is not the same as for the vegetarian East Indian. However, knowing your ancestry alone is not of much practical value, for it has become apparent that children from the same parents may not only differ to the extreme in external appearances and personalities, but also in terms of their nutritional requirements. This is particularly true of our modern society in America, which today is a genetic melting pot of the world.

However, the fact that your inherited nutritional requirements may be a matter of genetic roulette does not diminish the imperative need to meet those requirements. The bottom line still is that in order to be healthy, you *must* supply the body with all the raw materials, vitamins, minerals, and enzymes for which it has a genetic need. The failure to do so results in inefficiency of function of cells, organs, glands, and systems, imbalance in body chemistry, and eventually medically diagnosable dis-ease [sic].

Obviously, every vitamin and mineral is vital and necessary, but different people need *different amounts of the different nutrients*. Amazing as it may seem, it is very likely that most of the books touting the various nutrients are correct. *However, the books are accurate only for certain specific metabolic types; their recommendations are incorrect for other metabolic types!* This is what has made the field of nutrition so confusing.

What is an even more remarkable discovery now expounded by HEALTHEXCEL is that not only do different people need different amounts of nutrients, but also *any given nutrient can have an opposite reaction in different people. This explains why what improves one person's condition can actually worsen the same condition in someone else.* This discovery—that the way any given nutrient affects an individual depends upon the metabolic type of that individual—must be taken into account or any research experiments regarding the effects of nutrients will be quite meaningless.

This important understanding has yet another implication: *Any given health problem cannot be successfully addressed by a symptom-treatment approach.* To illustrate, consider the common problem of leg cramps. Leg cramps usually are an indication of a disruption of calcium metabolism. The common solution is to take additional calcium, and indeed for some metabolic types this is an effective and proper solution. But, few people realize that in other metabolic types this course of action provides not a solution but rather a worsening of the problem. For these metabolic types what is needed is not the ingestion of more calcium, but rather a diminishment of dietary calcium and an increase of those nutrients that are the biochemical "opposite," such as potassium and magnesium, in order to improve the utilization of calcium.

The principle illustrated with this relatively simple health adversity holds true for most all health problems as well. In order to successfully deal with an adverse health situation, it is imperative that you first understand the metabolic type in question before any recommendations are made. Only in this way can you be assured of getting your "medicine" and not your "poison." *The answer to the question regarding proper nutrition for any individual can only be obtained once the metabolic type of the individual is understood.*

The HEALTHEXCEL System

Through the HEALTHEXCEL System of Metabolic Typing, the clouds of confusion may be dispelled by providing a scientific (i.e., systematic, testable, repeatable, and verifiable) answer to the question regarding what you can do in order to be healthy. More than seven years of empirical research into the relationship of metabolic typing to the determination of individual nutritional requirements has uncovered a common denominator to all the systems of metabolic evaluation: energy! This realization has led to the further discovery that the previous systems of evaluation developed by the pioneers of metabolic nutritional research are in themselves neither right nor wrong, but are instead pieces of the same puzzle that complement rather than oppose each other.

Genes dictate the characteristics of each individual cell—the structure and purpose of the cell, the rate of cellular activity, the nutrients required by the cell for repairing and rebuilding, for reproduction, for energy production, and for successful completion of all cellular activities. Cells group together based upon similar makeup and purpose to form organs, glands, and other bodily tissues. These, in turn, form the various systems in the body whose purposes are to perform the special functions of the digestive system, the immune system, and so forth.

Metabolic Typing: Understanding Body Language

The HEALTHEXCEL System of Metabolic Typing is a process of evaluation of the interrelationship of the body's three main systems for the creation, maintenance, and control of energy: the autonomic nervous system, the oxidative system, and the endocrine system.

The nutrients obtained by the body from air, food, water, and light provide the fuel for all the processes of metabolism. By supplying the body with all the raw materials for which it has a genetic requirement, you set the stage for optimum energy production, the essential ingredient for good health and well-being.

Every activity in the body, whether it be physiological, psychological, or biochemical in nature, depends on the rate, quality, and amount of energy available. When the mind is clear and sharp, there is ample energy for emotional experience, and physical energy abounds. All the body's cells, organs, glands, and systems function efficiently and harmoniously. An overall feeling of vitality and well-being naturally pervades your experience.

But when the cells are deficient in their fuel requirements, and metabolic activity becomes disrupted, imbalanced, and inefficient, then the quality of your experience on all levels reflects that condition. The body then begins to communicate in its own "language" the fact that all is not well!

At first, it might just appear as a lessening of energy, of mental sharpness, or of emotional interest. Then actual non-specific symptoms or conditions, which are undiagnosable as an actual disease process, may begin to appear—such as headaches, digestive disturbances, constipation, food sensitivities; emotional disruptions, such as anger, irritability, depression for no apparent reason; apathy, lethargy, loss of interest in life, weight problems, loss of sex drive, disruption of energy levels, and so forth. If not corrected, such biochemical deficiencies may eventually give way to a full-blown, diagnosable degenerative disease.

But, long before that time, the body will have been communicating in its own fashion the fact that all is not well. The interpretation and the understanding of this body language is the quest of metabolic typing. In its own way, the body constantly defines its individuality; it gives expression to its imbalances and makes known the need for its requirements. The mental, emotional, and physical characteristics the body displays supply an ample description and unending flow of information regarding its status quo. You need only develop an understanding of the principles involved in metabolic typing in order to begin to understand the language of the body.

This understanding is effectively accomplished through HEALTHEXCEL's H.O.P.E. Survey (Health Optimization

Profile Evaluation): a 1,000-question computerized analysis that seeks an understanding of the physiological basis for the numerous and varied characteristics that comprise your individual metabolic experience. Understanding the physiological basis for all your characteristics allows for a categorization of all the known characteristics. Then, overall metabolic patterns and styles of functioning may be seen and the metabolic classification may be determined, based upon the three main energy systems of the body: the autonomic, oxidative, and endocrine systems. Once this is accomplished, nutritional recommendations in terms of diet and supplementation appropriate for your unique metabolic requirements can be made.

Then, by eating the very best organic foods *that are correct for your metabolic type,* by taking nutritional supplements *that are suitable for your nutritional individuality,* by avoiding toxins in your food and in your environment, by having regular structural treatments, and by cleansing and detoxifying your body regularly, you can truly make headway on the road to your optimal health and well-being!

Information About HEALTHEXCEL

HEALTHEXCEL, Inc., based in the foothills of the North Cascades in Eastern Washington State, is an education and information service company. Working through an established and growing referral network of health professionals, including medical doctors, dentists, osteopaths, chiropractors, nutritional consultants, and other health-related professionals, HEALTHEXCEL provides important information concerning individual nutritional requirements gleaned from complex and comprehensive computerized evaluation procedures.

Professionals employing the HEALTHEXCEL program in their practice can receive additional information and guidance by telephone from 10:00 a.m. to 10:00 p.m., Pacific time. Discussions center around the 100-page reports provided by HEALTHEXCEL as a result of the evaluation procedure, which includes valuable information about individual nutritional requirements. Extensive information is provided concerning each person's metabolic type, supplement recommendations, which foods are most appropriate for the individual's metabolism as well as why those foods are recommended and how they will effect one's metabolism.

If you decide that you would like to know more about metabolic typing, or what it would entail to find out about your unique nutritional requirements, you are invited to call or write to HEALTHEXCEL at the following address:

HEALTHEXCEL, Inc.,
Route 1, Box 495,
Winthrop, WA 98862.
Telephone: (509) 996-2131.

Printed by permission of William W. Wolcott.

12

Articles by Other Authors

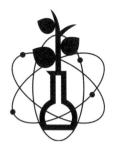

High-Colonic Irrigation

by Carol Signorella

Suppose you've jogged, dieted, gulped your vitamins, yet still feel fagged out and frail. This writer despaired of ever being jazzily vital, until she rediscovered a decades-old method of releasing natural energy . . .

"Colonic what?" I exclaimed.

"Colonic irrigation," Connie explained. "Like an internal bath to wash the poisons out of your system. You already know about all the unwanted food additives in our diets, and just think of the little extras not listed on the label. The pesticides sprayed on your fruits and vegetables, the hormones and antibiotics fed your beef and poultry. And then, if you want to talk about pollution. . . ."

"All right, Connie. So what happens when you're irrigated?"

"Simplicity itself. Water—tap water, usually—is slowly pumped up into the colon, our large intestine."

"An enema," I shuddered.

"In a way. But more water—an average of 25 to 30 gallons— is used and, under gentle pressure, it travels and cleanses the length of your colon, washing out all the stale bile and putrified waste poisoning your system. A colonic only takes an hour and is completely painless. You might even sleep through it."

Hmmmm, not likely, I thought. Still I had to admit that Connie's appearance had certainly improved since her first colonic irrigation three months before. Her eyes, skin, and hair all glowed. In fact, it's hard to describe Connie without making her sound like an ad for Short & Sassy.

That evening on the subway (where I do most of my serious thinking), I tallied my complaints: burning, itching eyes; yellow, dull skin; depression; anxiety; muddled head, uncoordinated body. Energy plummeted to a dreary low. For years I'd been busily trying out every possible cure for my persistent physical/emotional malaise; I'd jogged, quit smoking and drinking, added bran and dried fruit to my diet, even experimented with megavitamin therapy, but all to little avail. I remained dragged out, anxious, and definitely not my most vital self!

Why give up now? I thought. Maybe colonics could be a solution. Still, I wasn't going to let Connie talk me into anything without doing some independent research first. Naturally enough, I started with the American Medical Association—they, however, were less than helpful: "The AMA," I was told, "has no definitive statement on colonic irrigations; we neither recommend them nor are against them." A trip to the library at Columbia University College for Physicians and Surgeons proved equally unenlightening; their latest text on colonics was a 1927 volume titled *Troubles We Don't Talk About*.

The first professional opinion I sought also proved to be discouraging. My internist, Dr. Richard Nachtigall, who has a thriving Park Avenue practice, advised me to forget colonics. "I can't see much use for these irrigations," he said. "I've never heard of any real proof that they are useful except for certain abnormal conditions such as a defective liver, where it is necessary to remove bacteria-producing toxins." Dr. Milton Brothers, husband of Dr. Joyce Brothers, was even more emphatic: "I would never recommend them. It's an archaic practice and could be harmful. Colonics may induce a condition called electrolyte depletion. The bowel needs certain electrolytes—essential salts, acids, and alkalis—to perform its functions properly, and this sort of intensive irrigation could deplete the colon of these substances."

Not yet entirely deterred, I consulted another physician who believed colonics could improve health. "Nobody is really certain," he said, "where those all-important electrolytes are conserved, nor can any certain case be made for irrigation affecting their presence in the colon." Admitting that he personally believed in colonics (without including them in his practice), he also told me that these treatments are very popular among the rich and celebrated on the West Coast and in Europe. "Of course, it's just not something people want to talk about much," he explained, and then asked me to keep his name confidential. My anonymous source did, however, refer me to a Manhattan chiropractor and physical therapist who regularly performs this procedure, Dr. H. William Baum.

Dr. Baum, whose spritely step and taut, satinlike complexion belie his 85 years, practices naturopathic medicine; that is, he treats sickness primarily through natural means, believing that drugs and surgery should be resorted to only in extreme cases. Taking the holistic approach to health, the naturopath views disease not as an isolated malfunction, but rather as an indication that the entire body is in a state of "dis-ease."

For over 60 years, Dr. Baum has been performing colonic irrigations and has never found them less than effective and safe. I mentioned the negative views of the physicians I'd consulted, but Dr. Baum remained unfazed. "Most doctors don't prescribe vitamins, either," he said, sensibly enough. Reassured by Dr. Baum's manner and remembering the glow colonics had brought to my friend Connie, I swallowed hard and asked to be treated.

The first step was familiar enough; I changed into a pair of paper slippers and one of those thin, hospital-green gowns that open at the back. Then, clutching a pamphlet about colonics, I climbed aboard the long leather table and lay down on my side. The rectal applicator was inserted and the irrigation process began.

Throughout the colonic, I was attached to what resembled an old-fashioned water cooler, about four feet high and placed on the end of the examining table. When Dr. Baum pulled a lever in one direction, water burst into the clean, glass tank until it reached halfway to the top. Then the lever was reversed, and water began to slowly feed into me. The doctor moderated the pressure so that the water slowly worked its way through the twists and turns, obstructions and gases of the long large intestine.

After awhile, I realized with something like amazement that the water slushing up my intestinal tract had risen to just under my rib cage. Even so, I felt relaxed and experienced no pain. Dr. Baum's irrigation was much less unpleasant than either a home or hospital enema. I was not relaxed enough to drift right off to sleep, but I felt sufficiently comfortable to chat with Dr. Baum and learn a bit more about how and why colonics work. . . .

The indigestible portion of the food you eat, Dr. Baum explained, lodges in the large intestine and stays there until eliminated in a bowel movement. Infrequent movements or periods of constipation can, however, result in a partial decomposition of these waste substances that encrust the colon and further hinder elimination. These toxins are then reabsorbed into the bloodstream, lowering the body's defense against bacteria and viruses. The body strains to fight against the poisons and, if the effort is too great, various organs or even the circulatory system itself can break down. The early indications of this futile war against waste, Dr. Baum continued, include sallow skin, nervous irritability, coated tongue, bad breath, offensive body odor, headaches, bloating, poor appetite, and a feeling of stomach heaviness—symptoms that bore a marked resemblance to my own complaints.

Colonics might not be necessary, Dr. Baum went on, if

Americans had enough bulk in their diets, exercised regularly, and avoided alcohol, tobacco, polluted air, and processed foods. Few of us, however, do lead such uncontaminated lives.

Why, I wondered, can some people smoke and drink and eat poorly and still remain in good physical health? Dr. Baum explained that this lucky group has a tremendous natural capacity to eliminate toxins from their systems; but even so, he advised me not to be too jealous. "Their bad habits will catch up with them someday."

Colonic irrigations can be performed with varying frequency. Dr. Baum thinks first-time patients should have three in a row to be sure they're thoroughly cleansed, and after that, the number of treatments "depends on what I see coming out of you." A few people have one a week for years, others one a month, while most people are satisfied with three or four irrigations a year, often timing their treatments to correspond with the change of seasons.

"The shift to warm or cold weather," says Dr. Baum, "can upset the body's rhythms. An irrigation helps you adjust. Actually, these treatments aren't designed to cure any specific ailment; rather, they're designed to tune up the system so it becomes more capable of healing itself."

I asked Dr. Baum if a laxative would be equally effective. His answer was an emphatic no: "Colonics involve only the large intestine," he explained, "while laxatives pass through the small intestine as well. That's where digestion and absorption of nutrients occur, vital processes that should not be interfered with. Besides, emetics are, in a sense, addictive—for them to continue to be effective, you need to take larger doses."

So, with irrigation, the small intestine is left to itself (as it should be) and only the toxins contained in the colon are washed away. Dr. Baum's reasoning seemed sound enough to me as my hour-long irrigation drew to a close and I prepared to reap the benefits of his ministrations.

As I climbed off the treatment table, I felt wonderful—

high, energetic, positive, and strong. Before I left his office, Dr. Baum told me to take it easy the rest of the day and then suggested I change my diet to include lots of fresh fruits and vegetables, as well as plenty of bulk, and that I stay away from refined or processed foods. These changes would improve bowel functioning, he said, and lead to better overall health as well. I left feeling both peppy and inspired.

A few hours later, however, my high had completely faded, I was nauseous, dizzy, and nervously dialing Dr. Baum. He was not just reassuring, but positively congratulatory as I reeled off my symptoms. "That's the body continuing where the treatment left off," he told me. "The irrigation obviously stirred up a lot of poison. Eat something mild at regular intervals, rest, and come back in a few days for another treatment."

I did just that and continued the treatments once a month for nearly a year, sometimes adding an extra one when life was particularly stressful. I also followed Dr. Baum's advice about diet and within a few months noticed that I no longer had to discipline myself to eat properly. My craving for sugar had disappeared—I genuinely preferred an apple or helping of low-fat yogurt to a rich sweet. I also found myself developing a queasy aversion to coffee, cigarettes, and foods with preservatives—my body had learned to be naturally repelled by toxic substances.

After a year of colonics, my appearance and energy levels were both radically improved. No more draggy mornings or late-afternoon slumps. The bags under my eyes have disappeared entirely, and the sallow, yellowish tone that had spoiled my skin has been replaced by a healthy glow. I seem to think more clearly now, and I need less sleep. In a word, both my body and mind feel marvelously clean.

I couldn't be more enthusiastic about colonics.

Reprinted from *Cosmopolitan Magazine.*

Colonic Irrigation

by Angela Bell

The body comes into this world already knowing how to function in harmony—if its natural healing mechanisms are not interfered with. No one needs to teach a baby how to nurse or perform basic life processes of breathing, digestion, and elimination.

If the basic life processes somehow get out of balance, our inner environment can become a breeding ground for disease. Disease is not something that attacks us from without; it thrives in a mental and physical environment of lowered resistance that we allow.

If we neglect the body by feeding it improperly, failing to cleanse it inside or out, or treating it with disdain, we begin to create an inner environment where disease can flourish. The physical system then begins to rebel. In every way possible it tries to tell us to stop and evaluate our actions and thoughts—just as a true and loving friend might. Very often the body signals us with minor but annoying physical symptoms; these are not the disease, but only the outer signs of an imbalanced inner process.

Most of us never pay attention to these little warnings until we come down with a major dis-ease [sic]; then comes the mad race to eliminate symptoms (instead of the causes of disease). Unfortunately, this is not real healing. One of the warnings manifests as improper digestion and elimination.

Digestion is a multifaceted process. As food is taken into the mouth, the inner organs start a beautiful rhythmic dance. The esophagus moves rhythmically in a peristaltic action and moves the food into the stomach; the stomach begins its dance and then pushes the food into the small intestine. The small intestine begins its peristaltic movement, and thousands of tiny villi absorb the nutrients needed by the body and carry them into the bloodstream. (The villi also hold and later expel what the body does not need and cannot absorb.)

In a healthy person, the ileocecal valve opens and lets pass the waste that the small intestine has filtered out. Then, countless nerves are alerted to action, and this five-and-a-half foot organ rhythmically begins to push waste from the lower right side of the abdomen upward past the liver. At this point, the intestine turns across to the spleen, where it turns again, and then travels down to the floor of the pelvis, where it empties.

This process should occur every time we eat. The person who does not eliminate after every meal is constipated. If this occurs, the body begins to reabsorb its own waste and this situation provides an environment where disease can flourish.

Over a period of time, if the colon loses its ability to have a regular, rhythmic peristaltic flow, its nerve signals stop functioning and large deposits of waste gradually lodge in its many pockets and convolutions. This waste paralyzes the ileocecal valve, backs up into the small intestine, and is reabsorbed into the bloodstream. Parasites as well as bacteria flourish in this environment. Once the colon's flexures (turns) are plugged, it cannot support peristaltic action; it loses its "memory" and no longer functions in a healthy way.

Several things may cause the colon to "freeze" and its contents to back up:

1. Emotional stress may cause a tightening of the solar plexus nerve centers, inhibiting proper breathing and thus the flow of energy into the colon.

2. Improper dietary habits: white flour, devitalized or preserved foods, too much meat, spices, sugar, milk products; certain food allergies, etc.

3. Mental stress, mostly subconscious; previous poor toilet training, negative attitudes or anxiety about one's body functions.

These problems can be remedied without dependence on habit-forming laxatives. One solution is colonics.

Colonic irrigation is a cleansing process that uses a special machine to introduce warm water to the entire colon. Colonics are a safe, rapid way of unplugging the body's sewage system when it is no longer working effectively.

Colonic irrigation cannot be compared to an enema; it functions in a different manner. Enemas only empty the lower 12 inches of the five-and-a-half foot colon. The colonic irrigation reaches the entire length of the colon to the ileocecal valve; water flows out at the same rate it flows in. The process is painless, pleasant, and highly effective. It can remove the cause of chronic constipation and other diseases of the colon. The action of the water flowing in and being very gently drawn out through a very mild vacuum reminds the colon how to function on its own.

Once the colon regains its memory, it knows how to eliminate properly and no longer needs treatment. It does not need constant enemas to empty it; these tend to stretch and distort the lower rectal area of the colon and deaden the evacuation nerve impulses.

Once the colon is unblocked, self-maintenance is possible. We can keep our physical and mental channels open in a number of ways.

1. The solar plexus area is the only part of the body that is not covered by a bony structure. This is the center of your emotions. No creator would leave us without a way to keep this area clear; we can do it through the breath. Try this: lie down, relax as much as you can, and breathe from the diaphragm. Take in a breath and let everything out from the diaphragm. This will begin to allow energy to start to flow into that area; try to keep your mind only on your breathing. Even if you do this only five minutes a day, it will be beneficial; this type of breathing will also help tone the colon. At this time, you could also gently massage the colon from right to left. Breath is the first basic step to health.

2. Change your diet to a more natural one; stop eating the things that harm the body. Be kind to yourself. Feed yourself life-giving foods. Drink pure water. Educate yourself about nutrition. Nourishment is the second basic step to health.

3. Change your attitudes. Work with yourself. Be aware of how you feel about your own elimination processes. Love each thing about yourself. Don't put yourself down. Re-educate and reprogram yourself positively. In this physical world, your body is the house you live in; be comfortable in it. Accept it lovingly.

Clean the inner environment physically, emotionally, and mentally; no disease can flourish in a purified temple. In that type of environment, only the beauty of your own spirit and soul will grow.

Angela Bell is a licensed massage therapist who utilizes a holistic approach in her treatments. She also specializes in "Innerphasing," a reducing process that changes dietary habits.

Reprinted from *Alternatives Magazine*, January 1978.

Psychology of the Colon

by John Harvey Kellogg, M.D.

The colon is richly supplied with nerves and is highly sensitive to influence by all emotions pleasurable or the opposite. Studies have shown that unpleasant emotions of all sorts can stop peristalsis. Even very slight emotional excitement, such as slight anxiety, annoyance, apprehension, or ill-temper may stop all movement of the intestines, as well as of the stomach, together with gastric secretions.

The colon, like the face, responds to every passing emotion. The intestines are perhaps more sensitive than are the muscles of the face to emotional excitement because they are more richly supplied with blood vessels and sympathetic nerves.

X-ray studies of animals have demonstrated the intimate association of the colon with the sympathetic nervous system and the profound effects of all forms of emotional excitement. When a dog was placed in strange surroundings, peristalsis within its colon ceased for several hours. When a cat, while under observation, had its tail pinched, peristalsis also ceased. The movements did not begin again until the cat was pacified and purring contentedly.

The depressing influence of fear is well established. The frightened colon cannot discharge its contents because the descending colon is in a spastic state. So long as the patient is fearful that his bowels will not move, they will not. The colon is in a state of stage fright. It is crippled; but all that is needed for a cure may be to get rid of apprehension and fear. In such a case, the most effective remedies will not move the bowels until the element of fear is removed. Confidence and faith can change the situation.

The angry colon shuts up like a clam and declares "no thoroughfare here." Some persons are obstinately constipated because of a chronic state of ill will or anger.

Grief shuts up the outlet of the body's sewage system as tightly as does fear or anger. The worried colon neither secretes nor contracts. Both secretion and contraction are needed for efficient action—secretion for lubrication and contraction for transportation of the food residues to the exit. Loss of sleep, business worries, domestic trials, or harassment from any cause may render the colon dysfunctional.

In view of these facts, which might be multiplied at great length, it is evident that a right mental attitude as well as roughage and lubrication are essential for the successful treatment of a sluggish colon. With the laxative diet and various food accessories might be mingled the firm faith that the natural and biologic means employed will accomplish the desired outcome.

Such a faith will lead to regular visits to the toilet at the times when the bowels should move; that is, after each meal, on rising in the morning, and on going to bed at night. Do not wait for a "call," but invite a call by giving the colon a chance for evacuation and, by all means, avoid haste. A hurried visit to the toilet will not encourage normal colon activity. A slow colon must be given time, especially when by a change of diet and attention to colon hygiene it is just beginning to behave in something like a normal manner. By patient training, the sluggish bowel may after a time be trained to act with normal promptness and celerity.

From early infancy, the habit of prompt attention to the "call" for evacuation of the colon should be assiduously cultivated. Instead of doing this, the child is usually subjected to a process of housebreaking much like that to which house dogs are subjected. The result is the derangement of the natural order that empties the colon after each meal or three or four times a day. This establishes a crippled condition of the colon that permits but one evacuation a day, a form of constipation that is so universal among civilized people that it has come to be regarded as natural.

As soon as the child begins to run about, the mother begins to train him to restrain the movements of his bladder and bowels to suit convenience of time and place. A false sense of modesty also becomes a restraining influence that soon upsets the normal intestinal rhythm and lays the foundation for lifelong constipation and all the miseries associated with these conditions and the autointoxication to which they give rise.

Indeed, the majority of people and many physicians regard regularity as the essential element of colon health, and almost ignore the matter of frequency and thoroughness of evacuation. The late Sir Lauder Brunton, an eminent English internist, told of a lady who answered his inquiry about her colon function, "Perfectly regular, sir, perfectly regular." When further questioned, she disclosed the fact that although bowel movements were perfectly regular, they occurred only once in three weeks.

This article contains excerpts from Dr. John Harvey Kellog's writing on colon health (1928). Dr. Kellog founded the Battle Creek, Michigan, Sanitarium and the Kellogg's Breakfast Cereal Company.

Colon Therapy: The Natural Way to Renewed Health

by Sheila Shea

We are all trained from early childhood to have very negative attitudes toward our organs of elimination. The colon and the anus are still taboo topics and people are not educated to treat their organs with care and respect.

Like millions of others who neglect their colons, I suffered through the years from chronic constipation, discomfort, and poor health. The constant muscle tensions were distorting my personality, and the accumulated toxins were poisoning my body, but all these problems were cleared up after I began the regular practice of watching my diet and cleansing my colon.

Actually, I was forced to confront my own digestive tract because I watched others in my family succumb to colon disorders. My father had cancer of the colon, my grandmother had severe intestinal problems, and my mother has been constipated much of her life. So, after I had undergone colonic therapy for a while, I decided to become a colon therapist. Now I have the continuing satisfaction of helping many people who suffer from distress of this vital organ.

A colonic is a gentle, warm-water washing of the colon or large intestine, combined with an external massage. At the foot of the massage table is a colon irrigation machine, which is simply a tank with tubing and a few levers and valves. One end of the tubing is put gently into the rectum.

Water flows into the colon, and when the client feels any pressure or discomfort, he or she asks for release. This process of filling and releasing is repeated until the colon is emptied. If desired, the contents of the colon may be viewed as they flow through a glass tube on their way to the drain.

A colonic usually lasts 45 minutes to an hour. While the water is leaving the colon, the irrigationist gives an abdominal massage in patterns to help eliminate gas, fecal matter, and mucous.

Most people are able to cleanse only about half of the colon by themselves via enemas. But, for a thorough cleansing of the entire colon—a high colonic—it is best to have the services of an experienced therapist.

My first introduction to colon irrigation came through Norman Walker's book *Raw Vegetable Juices,* and the works of natural healer Arnold Ehret. Both authors believe that constipation is a basic cause of disease that can be remedied by dissolving the backlog of toxins and mucous. I began increasing my intake of citrus and vegetable juices to dissolve the mucous, but it wasn't until I was 31 that I had my first colon irrigation. I think I resisted getting one because I felt terribly ashamed of my chronic constipation. Also, from years of straining and resultant hemorrhoids, I had a very finnicky, sensitive anus, and I didn't like the thought of inserting anything into it.

However, a very close friend of mine had received a series of colonics and had encouraged me to do it, too. So we went to the Hippocrates Health Institute in Boston, and tried their diet of raw foods and vegetable juices for two weeks.

I still resisted the idea of a colonic, but my friend offered to go with me. As the institute's therapist began the colonic I burst into tears. My anal muscles were as tight as my jaw and neck muscles, and it was a truly emotional experience to try to loosen them. But I made it through the session and came back the next week for another—and they got easier and better as I became more accustomed to them.

Mine was an extreme case of dysfunction. In addition to my general physical problems, sex was often unpleasant for me.

The Colon Is a Neighbor

The colon lives in very close quarters with the kidneys, ovaries, bladder, and uterus or prostate gland. Roommates, if you will. In my case I had complaints ranging from vaginal infections and cystitis to herpes. Never once did I consider that any of these problems related were to my colon.

I had been constipated for the first 26 years of life until I began taking enemas, a simple water cleansing of the colon using a standard two-quart bag. As I continued to cleanse my colon on a regular basis with colonics, fasting, raw juices, and more live foods, all of the symptoms of these infections disappeared and to this date have not returned.

You see, when the colon does not release its contents on a regular basis, the backlog of fecal matter putrefies. This putrefaction occurs through bacterial action. These bacteria multiply very rapidly and can pass through the walls of the colon to other organs. The bacteria begin the same process on these organs, which is to break down their proper function.

These bacteria create strong acids and gases that cause inflammation. They are ultimately released via the urethra or vaginal canal in the form of mucous or pus. The foods that these pathogenic or harmful bacteria thrive on are animal products, sugar, dairy, drugs, and chemicals.

When the slightest symptoms of these basic infections appear, the first thing to do is cleanse the colon and check your diet. If you have been indulging in any of the main offenders, lay off them. If your diet has been quite clean, then you are experiencing a cleansing of older material, remnants of that old diet of meat, dairy, sugar, salt, flour, and you know the rest.

I have also found that by adding a living primary yeast to my diet, I can minimize an infection to seven days and at the same time rejuvenate my immune system. I also suggest increasing the intake of green vegetables and fresh fruit. Harmful bacteria cannot thrive in an environment of greens and fruit.

All of the organs of the abdominal area are beautiful neighbors. It is a small but important community where cooperation, harmony, cleanliness, and comfort are of paramount value in maintaining and improving the quality of your health.

Focusing awareness and attention on the state of your colon is not only good hygiene and the prelude to natural healing—it is also an ancient form of yogic meditation. According to the yogic system, the body has seven centers of energy, or chakras. Each is an important center of psychic and physical energy, and all must function harmoniously and without impediment for the body to experience optimum health and well-being.

These centers are located at the anus, the sex organs, the solar plexus, the heart, the throat, the place between and above the eyes, and the top of the head. When there is distress or blockage in any of these centers, the entire balance of the body is thrown off. Yogis give sober attention, care, and meditation to each center. They feel its state from within—whether it is tense or relaxed, functioning smoothly or paralyzed with blockage. Yogic exercises are very useful for toning the abdomen; they can also be practiced during colonics.

People have asked me if I think it's unnatural to take so many enemas and colonics. With my history of chronic constipation, I have never known what is "natural." I find taking salt, sugar, chemicals, drugs, alcohol, highly refined foods, and not exercising on a regular basis "unnatural" for my body now. I think it's more "natural" in this society to be constantly ill, in pain, and constipated.

As a practicing colonic therapist, I've been astounded at all the fear, guilt, and shame people have built up. They're afraid they will "dirty" the table (that's what it's for), and they're embarrassed to talk about the process of elimination. The blackout in this culture about the whole lowest chakra or energy center, the anus, is almost total. Since the anus is the base of energy, balance, pleasure, power and security, to be constipated is literally to be "up tight."

Clients come to me for colon irrigation for many reasons: constipation, gas, sciatic pains, rheumatoid arthritis, cleansing to accompany diets, fasting, and pregnancy, cleansing before sex or an artistic performance, headaches (especially migraine), worms, after binges, in combination with diet change and weight loss, to combat poisoning from excess refined sugar, flour, and predigested animal protein—in short, for all problems caused by an overload of toxins in the body.

A few people come in tense, very hyper from the day's activities. Others talk compulsively on the table. Many try to hold back. In each case, the person has an inability to focus on his or her body and its physical functions. I tell each of them that colon irrigation is a meditation for the colon and that any kind of release is okay.

One potential client told me she was afraid to come in because of what I would see in the viewing tube. She wanted to get herself "clean" before she came in because she was afraid I would judge her and say her diet was bad and therefore she was bad. This is like cleaning house before your maid arrives, so she won't have a low opinion of your character.

Too many of my clients either hold in or push when they feel the pleasurable wave of release. Both actions constrict all the muscles in the lower pelvic bowel and prevent a cleansing. I call this reaction pleasure anxiety, and I teach people to let go of the closed-off sigmoid colon. Training people in the pleasure of releasing is part of a colonic therapist's job. I have achieved many breakthroughs using breathing, meditation, focus, massage, and water!

The factors that make cleansings more difficult are a prolapsed or fallen transverse colon; enlarged, impacted gas pockets; too much or too little muscle tone; a weak sigmoid colon; pushing or straining at the stool; and drugs that inhibit the colon.

Most people—including myself—have a prolapsed transverse colon.* The transverse has fallen like a hammock, usually to a point somewhere below the navel. The transverse then

---

*See page 41 for diagram.

falls on other organs, such as the bladder or uterus, which in turn fall on the sigmoid colon and close it off.

Some causes of a prolapsed transverse colon are engorging the stomach with too much food, weak muscle tone from toxic diets and lack of exercise, poor posture, and impacted pockets. There is a continuous series of one-to-two-inch pockets or saculations along the colon. These pockets enlarge when solids collect in them and are not eliminated. Decomposing meat and starches can even harden on the wall and cause a pocket to become impacted. When solids get stuck in the pockets, they putrefy or rot, creating more toxic wastes and gas, which expand the pockets further. I've had some marvelous results working out the contents of the pockets using various massage techniques. Abdominal massage is something you can do for yourself any time you want to loosen matter in the colon and stimulate peristalsis (alternating expansion and contraction of the entire digestive tube).

Most times gas is caused by improper food combinations, matter putrefying in pockets of the colon, mucous softening and being released from the colon wall, and inorganic toxic gases excreted by body cells.

The major improper combination is eating fruit or sugar with or after any starch, protein, or vegetable other than a green. When combined improperly, fruit, sugar, and alcohol ferment and cause gas, as well as expand gas that's already formed.

During a cleansing diet or a liquid fast, mucous is dislodged from the colon wall, often preceded by tremendous amounts of gas. Certain natural foods high in sulphur or chlorine, such as avocado or members of the cabbage family, release toxic gases by replacing them with natural ones. The gases are released more heavily when a person begins a natural food diet or a fast.

It is important to get gas out of the colon. As well as serving as a conduit for food wastes, the colon eliminates wastes from blood, lymph, liver, and nervous systems. When the colon is not being emptied regularly, these toxins are reabsorbed into the blood and nerves.

Drugs may also have an inhibiting effect on the colon. For example, antibiotics destroy the natural flora that live there and aid digestion. Certain chemicals, salts, and sugars in the diet have the same effect. Flora are not drawn from the colon wall with a water cleansing, but one candy bar wipes them out! Fresh fruit and vegetables, fermented foods, and unpasteurized yogurt and acidophilus continue to provide the colon with fresh flora.

A highly refined diet of salts, sugars, flours, fats, and dairy products causes mucous to harden on the walls of the colon. Although the body needs high-quality mucous in it at all times as a natural lubricant, "good" mucous has a liquid consistency and is derived from a diet of whole foods.

Good muscle tone in the abdomen is also essential for healthy elimination. Sometimes the abdominal muscles are overly tight from psychological tension or the wrong kind of abdominal exercises. Surgery can cause holding patterns in the muscles, also producing too much tension.

However, it is lack of muscle tone that is most common. When muscle tone is correct, involuntary contractions move solids, liquids, and gases rhythmically from one part of the body to the other.

For most people, gravity moves material through the colon. More input pushes what is already there a little bit farther down. Diet, exercise, and breathing—along with colonics or enemas—begin to stimulate peristalsis by breaking up large pockets of gas and impacted matter, loosening mucous, and toning abdominal muscles.

All in all, the benefits of high-colonic sessions are exercise of the rectal muscles, release of abdominal tension, the flushing out of accumulated toxins, and the relief of gas pains. Also, colon irrigation provides a chance for a person to take a break from his or her normal consciousness and focus on the true center of personal power—the colon. Restoring it to strong peristalsis, good tone, and harmonious functioning has a beneficial effect on your state of mind, your health, and your sex life.

Sheila Shea, D.D., is a Miami-based colon irrigationist who since 1970 has been devoted to self-healing and research on the colon.

Reprinted from *Forum Magazine: The Journal of Human Relations*, Forum International, Ltd., 1978.

13

Quotes from America's Leading Experts on Colon Health

The Doctor
of the Future
Will give no medicine
But will interest his
Patient in the care of
The human frame, in diet,
And in the cause
And prevention of disease.
　　　　—Thomas A. Edison

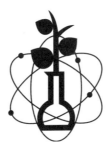

Quotes from Bernard Jensen, D.C., Ph.D.

- It's often said that you are what you eat. I say that you are what you absorb.
- Insufficient numbers of bowel movements and too little fiber and bulk in the feces may often explain the existence of gall bladder disorders, heart problems, varicose veins, appendicitis, clotting in deep veins, hiatal hernia, diverticulosis, arthritis, and cancer of the colon.
- To try to take care of any symptom in the body without a good elimination is futile.
- I believe autointoxication is currently the number one source of the misery and decay we are witnessing in our society and culture today.
- The road to health is the one that begins with an understanding and commitment to cleanse and detoxify the body, to restore balance, peace, and harmony.
- The greatest healing power comes from within out.
- It takes an extreme measure of action and courage in order to get out of the bowel situation in which so many people find themselves. Knowing the ways of keeping the bowel healthy and in good shape is the best way I know to keep away from the grip of disease and sickness.
- The bowel-wise person is the one who is armed with good knowledge, practices discrimination in his eating habits, and walks the path of higher life. His days are blessed with

health, vitality, optimism, and the fulfillment of life's goals. He is a blessing and source of inspiration to family associates. His cheerful disposition comes from having a vital, toxin-free body made possible by the efficient, regular cleansing action of a loved and well-cared-for bowel.

Bernard Jensen, D.C., Ph.D.

Quotes reprinted by permission of Bernard Jensen, D.C., Ph.D.

Quotes from Norman Walker, D.Sc.

- Colon health emphasizes prevention rather than cure. It is the most important step in maintaining or regaining vital health.
- Colon irrigation along with other health programs have kept me ageless. No matter what—colon cleansings don't hurt you, they can only help you. If you think about it, they make sense.
- Most health enthusiasts don't realize that the colon is responsible for the assimilation of minerals and vitamins. Supplements at best are only partially absorbed with a clogged, encrusted, or heavily coated colon.
- Overweight is often the result of a backed-up system. Food stores rather than metabolizes.
- The hardened material that accumulates on the inside walls of the colon is like cement. It does not come down by itself, or with fasts, laxatives, enemas, or drugs, and it is at the root of many human problems.
- If the sewer system in your home is backed up, your entire home is affected. Should it be any different with your body?
- Don't just wait until your colon is completely blocked. Always think in terms of prevention. More than one million victims [of colon surgery] spent more than two billion dollars for surgery and convalescence, and that's only the beginning.
- The colon, just like the spine, is interrelated, interconnected, and interdependent with every other part of the body. Health in the colon often affects health in other areas of the body.
- Waste matter naturally collected in the colon and allowed to remain longer than necessary is by nature subject to fermentation and putrefaction, which is an area of toxicity

that can be picked up by the bloodstream and settle in any part of your body.

• Colon irrigations help chiropractic adjustments keep, because of the decreased toxicity level. There is an interrelationship, one compliments the other.

Norman W. Walker, D.Sc., as a centenarian

Quotes reprinted by permission of Norman W. Walker, D.Sc., from his book *Colon Health: The Key to a Vibrant Life* (Norwalk Press, Prescott, Arizona).

References and Suggested Reading

Abravanel, Elliot, M.D.
Body Type Diet

Bieler, Henry, M.D.
Food Is Your Best Medicine (Ballantine Books, 1965)

Brown, Thomas, M.D.
The Road Back (M. Evans & Company, 1988)

Burton, Gail
The Candida Control Cookbook (New American Library, 1989)

Connolly, Pat
The Candida Albicans Yeast Free Cookbook

Harrower, Henry
Practical Endocrinology

Jensen, Bernard, D.C., Ph.D.
Tissue Cleansing through Bowel Management
Foods that Heal (Avery Publications, 1988)
Love, Sex and Nutrition (Avery Publications, 1988)
Vibrant Health From Your Kitchen
Nature Has a Remedy
Herbal Handbook

Kelley, William D., D.D.S.
The Metabolic Types
One Answer to Cancer

Kellogg, John, M.D.
Autointoxication or Intestinal Toxemia (Modern
Medicine Publishing Company, 1922)

Kulvinskas, Viktoras
Life in the 21st Century (Omangod Press, 1981)

Pottenger, Francis M., M.D.
Symptoms of Visceral Disease

Rohe, Fred and Dr. William Kelley
Metabolic Ecology: A Way to Win the Cancer War
(Wedgestone Press, 1982)

Steinman, David
Diet for a Poisoned Planet (Harmony Books, 1990)

Tilden, J. H., M.D.
Toxemia Explained (Health Research, 1952)
*Appendicitis: The Etiology, Hygienic and Dietetic
Treatment* (Health Research, 1976)

Truss, C. Orian, M.D.
The Missing Diagnosis

Valentine, Tom & Carole
Metabolic Typing (Thorsons Publishing Group, 1986)

Walker, Norman, D.Sc.
Colon Health: The Key to a Vibrant Life (Norwalk Press)
Vibrant Health: The Possible Dream (Norwalk Press)
Raw Vegetable Juices (Norwalk Press, 1978)

Watson, George, Ph.D.
*Nutrition and Your Mind, Personality Strength
and Psychochemical Energy*

Williams, Roger, Ph.D.
Biochemical Individuality:, Nutrition Against Disease

Order Forms

Healing Within Products

P.O. Box 1013 • Larkspur, CA 94977-1013

Orders Only (800) 300-7548 • in Calif call (415) 454-6677 • Fax (415) 454-6659

effective 3/21/96

Healing Within Products Order Form

Prod. No.	• *Healing Within Complete Kits* •	Price
102	**4 to 7-Day Cleansing Kit (for all body weights)** .... Castor Oil (16 oz. liquid), Colon 8 Intestinal Cleanser (1 bottle, 120 caplets), DDS Acidophilus (1 bottle, 100 capsules), Dr. Jensen's Broth (5 oz.), Dry Skin Brush, Flannel Cloth, KB-11 (1 bottle, 60 tablets), OXY-OXC (1 bottle, 180 capsules), Pau D'Arco Tea (4 oz. bulk package), Whole Life Food Blend (16 oz. concentrate). **Total Products: 10 Items**	$129.00
	Each Kit Shipping, Handling & Insurance	8.00
101	**Candida Elimination Kit (for all body weights)** .... Arizona Natural Garlic (1 bottle, 250 capsules), Caprystatin (4 bottles, 90 tablets each), Colon 8 Intestinal Cleanser (2 bottles, 120 caplets each), Coenzyme Q10 (2 bottles, 50 capsules each, 30 mg.), DDS Acidophilus (3 bottles, 100 capsules each), Kaprycidin-A (2 bottles, 90 capsules each), Immuno-Quest (2 bottles, 100 capsules each), Natur-Earth (2 bottles, 90 capsules each), Orithrush-D (1 bottle, 8 fl. oz. concentrate), OXY-OXC (2 bottles, 180 capsules each), Pau D'Arco Tea (2 boxes, 4 oz. bulk package each), Travacid X (2 bottles, 100 caplets each), Dioxychlor DC-3 (2 bottles, 1 oz. each), Latero Flora (2 bottles, 60 capsules each). **Total Products: 29 Items**	$580.00
	Each Kit Shipping, Handling & Insurance	12.00
103	**Parasite Elimination Kit A1 (for body weight under 100 lbs.)** .. Black Walnut Tincture (1 bottle, 4 oz.), Castor Oil Capsules (2 bottles, 180 capsules each), DDS Acidophilus (2 bottles, 100 capsules each), Echinacea (2 bottles, 90 capsules each), Gozarte (3 bottles, 60 capsules each), Healing Within Intestinal Cleanser (2 bottles, 250 capsules each), Intestinalis Herbal Cleanser (1 bottle, 60 tablets), K-Min (2 bottles, 180 capsules each), Latero Flora (2 bottles, 60 capsules each), Shitake Mushrooms (2 bottles, 90 capsules each). **Total Products: 19 Items**	$529.00
	Each Kit Shipping, Handling & Insurance	12.00
104	**Parasite Elimination Kit A2 (for body weight under 100 lbs.)** .. Black Walnut Tincture (1 bottle, 4 oz.), Castor Oil Capsules (2 bottles, 180 capsules each), DDS Acidophilus (2 bottles, 100 capsules each), Echinacea (2 bottles, 90 capsules each), Healing Within Intestinal Cleanser (2 bottles, 250 capsules each), Intestinalis Herbal Cleanser (1 bottle, 60 tablets), K-Min (2 bottles, 180 capsules each), Latero Flora (2 bottles, 60 capsules each), Pasaloc (3 bottles, 60 capsules each), Shitake Mushrooms (2 bottles, 90 capsules each). **Total Products: 19 Items**	$529.00
	Each Kit Shipping, Handling & Insurance	12.00

Prod. No.	• *Healing Within Complete Kits* (cont.) •	Price
105	**Parasite Elimination Kit A3 (for body weight under 100 lbs.)** .. Black Walnut Tincture (1 bottle, 4 oz.), Castor Oil Capsules (2 bottles, 180 capsules each), DDS Acidophilus (2 bottles, 100 capsules each), Echinacea (2 bottles, 90 capsules each), Gozarte (3 bottles, 60 capsules each), Healing Within Intestinal Cleanser (2 bottles, 250 capsules each), Intestinalis Herbal Cleanser (1 bottle, 60 tablets), K-Min (2 bottles, 180 capsules each), Latero Flora (2 bottles, 60 capsules each), Neo-Pararte (3 bottles, 60 capsules each), Shitake Mushrooms (2 bottles, 90 capsules each). **Total Products: 22 Items**	$757.00
	Each Kit Shipping, Handling & Insurance	12.00
106	**Parasite Elimination Kit A4 (for body weight under 100 lbs.)** .. Black Walnut Tincture (1 bottle, 4 oz.), Castor Oil Capsules (2 bottles, 180 capsules each), DDS Acidophilus (2 bottles, 100 capsules each), Echinacea (2 bottles, 90 capsules each), Healing Within Intestinal Cleanser (2 bottles, 250 capsules each), Intestinalis Herbal Cleanser (1 bottle, 60 tablets), K-Min (2 bottles, 180 capsules each), Latero Flora (2 bottles, 60 capsules each), Padapco (3 bottles, 60 capsules each), Pasaloc (3 bottles, 60 capsules each), Shitake Mushrooms (2 bottles, 90 capsules each). **Total Products: 22 Items**	$757.00
	Each Kit Shipping, Handling & Insurance	12.00
106A	**Parasite Elimination Kit A5 (for body weight under 100 lbs.)** .. Black Walnut Tincture (1 bottle, 4 oz.), Castor Oil Capsules (2 bottles, 180 capsules each), DDS Acidophilus (2 bottles, 100 capsules each), Echinacea (2 bottles, 90 capsules each), Gozarte (3 bottles, 60 capsules each), Healing Within Intestinal Cleanser (2 bottles, 250 capsules each), Intestinalis Herbal Cleanser (1 bottle, 60 tablets), K-Min (2 bottles, 180 capsules each), Latero Flora (2 bottles, 60 capsules each), Shitake Mushrooms (2 bottles, 90 capsules each), Udarte (3 bottles, 60 capsules each). **Total Products: 22 Items**	$757.00
	Each Kit Shipping, Handling & Insurance	12.00
107	**Parasite Elimination Kit B1 (for body weight 100-175 lbs.)** .... Black Walnut Tincture (1 bottle, 4 oz.), Castor Oil Capsules (3 bottles, 180 capsules each), DDS Acidophilus (2 bottles, 100 capsules each), Echinacea (2 bottles, 90 capsules each), Gozarte (3 bottles, 60 capsules each), Healing Within Intestinal Cleanser (2 bottles, 250 capsules each), Intestinalis Herbal Cleanser (1 bottle, 60 tablets), K-Min (2 bottles, 180 capsules each), Latero Flora (2 bottles, 60 capsules each), Shitake Mushrooms (2 bottles, 90 capsules each). **Total Products: 20 Items**	$542.00
	Each Kit Shipping, Handling & Insurance	12.00
108	**Parasite Elimination Kit B2 (for body weight 100-175 lbs.)** .... Black Walnut Tincture (1 bottle, 4 oz.), Castor Oil Capsules (3 bottles, 180 capsules each), DDS Acidophilus (2 bottles, 100 capsules each), Echinacea (2 bottles, 90 capsules each), Healing Within Intestinal Cleanser (2 bottles, 250 capsules each), Intestinalis Herbal Cleanser (1 bottle, 60 tablets), K-Min (2 bottles, 180 capsules each), Latero Flora (2 bottles, 60 capsules each), Pasaloc (3 bottles, 60 capsules each), Shitake Mushrooms (2 bottles, 90 capsules each). **Total Products: 23 Items**	$542.00
	Each Kit Shipping, Handling & Insurance	12.00

Prod. No.	• *Healing Within Complete Kits* (cont.) •	Price
109	**Parasite Elimination Kit B3 (for body weight 100-175 lbs.)** .... Black Walnut Tincture (1 bottle, 4 oz.), Castor Oil Capsules (3 bottles, 180 capsules each), DDS Acidophilus (2 bottles, 100 capsules each), Echinacea (2 bottles, 90 capsules each), Gozarte (3 bottles, 60 capsules each), Healing Within Intestinal Cleanser (2 bottles, 250 capsules each), Intestinalis Herbal Cleanser (1 bottle, 60 tablets), K-Min (2 bottles, 180 capsules each), Latero Flora (2 bottles, 60 capsules each), Neo-Pararte (3 bottles, 60 capsules each), Shitake Mushrooms (2 bottles, 90 capsules each). **Total Products: 23 Items**	$770.00
	Each Kit Shipping, Handling & Insurance	12.00
110	**Parasite Elimination Kit B4 (for body weight 100-175 lbs.)** .... Black Walnut Tincture (1 bottle, 4 oz.), Castor Oil Capsules (3 bottles, 180 capsules each), DDS Acidophilus (2 bottles, 100 capsules each), Echinacea (2 bottles, 90 capsules each), Healing Within Intestinal Cleanser (2 bottles, 250 capsules each), Intestinalis Herbal Cleanser (1 bottle, 60 tablets), K-Min (2 bottles, 180 capsules each), Latero Flora (2 bottles, 60 capsules each), Padapco (3 bottles, 60 capsules each), Pasaloc (3 bottles, 60 capsules each), Shitake Mushrooms (2 bottles, 90 capsules each). **Total Products: 23 Items**	$770.00
	Each Kit Shipping, Handling & Insurance	12.00
110A	**Parasite Elimination Kit B5 (for body weight 100-175 lbs.)** .... Black Walnut Tincture (1 bottle, 4 oz.), Castor Oil Capsules (3 bottles, 180 capsules each), DDS Acidophilus (2 bottles, 100 capsules each), Echinacea (2 bottles, 90 capsules each), Gozarte (3 bottles, 60 capsules each), Healing Within Intestinal Cleanser (2 bottles, 250 capsules each), Intestinalis Herbal Cleanser (1 bottle, 60 tablets), K-Min (2 bottles, 180 capsules each), Latero Flora (2 bottles, 60 capsules each), Shitake Mushrooms (2 bottles, 90 capsules each), Udarte (3 bottles, 60 capsules each). **Total Products: 23 Items**	$770.00
	Each Kit Shipping, Handling & Insurance	12.00
111	**Parasite Elimination Kit C1 (for body weight over 175 lbs.)** ... Black Walnut Tincture (1 bottle, 4 oz.), Castor Oil Capsules (4 bottles, 180 capsules each), DDS Acidophilus (2 bottles, 100 capsules each), Echinacea (2 bottles, 90 capsules each), Gozarte (3 bottles, 60 capsules each), Healing Within Intestinal Cleanser (3 bottles, 250 capsules each), Intestinalis Herbal Cleanser (1 bottle, 60 tablets), K-Min (2 bottles, 180 capsules each), Latero Flora (2 bottles, 60 capsules each), Shitake Mushrooms (2 bottles, 90 capsules each). **Total Products: 22 Items**	$575.00
	Each Kit Shipping, Handling & Insurance	12.00
112	**Parasite Elimination Kit C2 (for body weight over 175 lbs.)** ... Black Walnut Tincture (1 bottle, 4 oz.), Castor Oil Capsules (4 bottles, 180 capsules each), DDS Acidophilus (2 bottles, 100 capsules each), Echinacea (2 bottles, 90 capsules each), Healing Within Intestinal Cleanser (3 bottles, 250 capsules each), Intestinalis Herbal Cleanser (1 bottle, 60 tablets), K-Min (2 bottles, 180 capsules each), Latero Flora (2 bottles, 60 capsules each), Pasaloc (3 bottles, 60 capsules each), Shitake Mushrooms (2 bottles, 90 capsules each). **Total Products: 22 Items**	$575.00
	Each Kit Shipping, Handling & Insurance	12.00

Prod. No.	• *Healing Within Complete Kits* (cont.) •	Price
113	**Parasite Elimination Kit C3 (for body weight over 175 lbs.)** ... Black Walnut Tincture (1 bottle, 4 oz.), Castor Oil Capsules (4 bottles, 180 capsules each), DDS Acidophilus (2 bottles, 100 capsules each), Echinacea (2 bottles, 90 capsules each), Gozarte (3 bottles, 60 capsules each), Healing Within Intestinal Cleanser (3 bottles, 250 capsules each), Intestinalis Herbal Cleanser (1 bottle, 60 tablets), K-Min (2 bottles, 180 capsules each), Latero Flora (2 bottles, 60 capsules each), Neo-Pararte (3 bottles, 60 capsules each), Shitake Mushrooms (2 bottles, 90 capsules each). **Total Products: 25 Items**	$803.00
	Each Kit Shipping, Handling & Insurance	12.00
114	**Parasite Elimination Kit C4 (for body weight over 175 lbs.)** ... Black Walnut Tincture (1 bottle, 4 oz.), Castor Oil Capsules (4 bottles, 180 capsules each), DDS Acidophilus (2 bottles, 100 capsules each), Echinacea (2 bottles, 90 capsules each), Healing Within Intestinal Cleanser (3 bottles, 250 capsules each), Intestinalis Herbal Cleanser (1 bottle, 60 tablets), K-Min (2 bottles, 180 capsules each), Latero Flora (2 bottles, 60 capsules each), Padapco (3 bottles, 60 capsules each), Pasaloc (3 bottles, 60 capsules each), Shitake Mushrooms (2 bottles, 90 capsules each). **Total Products: 25 Items**	$803.00
	Each Kit Shipping, Handling & Insurance	12.00
115	**Parasite Elimination Kit C5 (for body weight over 175 lbs.)** ... Black Walnut Tincture (1 bottle, 4 oz.), Castor Oil Capsules (4 bottles, 180 capsules each), DDS Acidophilus (2 bottles, 100 capsules each), Echinacea (2 bottles, 90 capsules each), Gozarte (3 bottles, 60 capsules each), Healing Within Intestinal Cleanser (3 bottles, 250 capsules each), Intestinalis Herbal Cleanser (1 bottle, 60 tablets), K-Min (2 bottles, 180 capsules each), Latero Flora (2 bottles, 60 capsules each), Shitake Mushrooms (2 bottles, 90 capsules each), Udarte (3 bottles, 60 capsules each). **Total Products: 25 Items**	$803.00
	Each Kit Shipping, Handling & Insurance	12.00
116	**Three Phase Intestinal Flora Rebuilding Program** .... **(for all body weights)** Replete (2 bottles, 7 powder sachets each), HMF Forte (2 bottles, 45 capsules each), HMF (2 bottles, 60 capsules each), Livit 2 (2 bottles, 90 tablets each), Whey Plex (2 bottles, 4 oz. powder each), Vyta Myns (2 bottles, 90 capsules each), Trifals, (2 bottles, 90 capsules each). **Total Products 14 Items.**	$368.00
	Each Kit Shipping, Handling & Insurance	10.00

Prod. No.	• *Healing Within Individual Items* •	Price
201	**Acidophilus, DDS, 100 capsules**	$ 17.00
202	**Acidophilus, HMF, 60 capsules**	24.00
203	**Acidophilus, Ultra-Probiotic, 1.75 oz.**	25.00
205	**Aloe-Ace Aloe Vera, 4 oz. concentrate (makes 1 gallon)**	25.00

Prod. No.	• *Healing Within Individual Items (cont.)*•	Price
206	Aloe-V, 450 mg., 100 caplets	$ 20.00
207	Arizona Natural Garlic, 250 capsules	14.00
314	Arthritis Care, 50 capsules	300.00
209	Black Walnut Tincture, 4 oz. Green Hulls	12.00
211	Caprastatin, 90 tablets	18.00
212	Castor Oil, 16 oz. liquid	12.00
213	Castor Oil Capsules, 180 capsules	13.00
214	Cats Claw, 350 mg., 90 capsules	17.00
280	Cats Claw, 4 oz. bulk tea	22.00
281	Cats Claw, 500 mg., 90 capsules	22.00
311	Clarkia 100, 2 fl. oz.	30.00
215	Coenzyme Q10, 60 capsules, 30 mg. each	27.00
282	Coenzyme Q10, 50 capsules, 30 mg. each	21.00
216	Col Verb-Q, 60 capsules	76.00
283	Colloidal Silver, 4 oz.	30.00
284	Consolar, 60 capsules	45.00
217	Coral Calcium, 30-day supply	35.00
219	Digestase, 90 capsules	24.00
220	Dioxychlor DC3, 1 oz.	26.00
222	Dr. Jensen's Broth, 5 oz.	5.00
223	Dry Skin Brush	6.00
224	Echinacea, 90 capsules	20.00
225	Ecomer, 60 capsules	20.00
221	Essiac Tea	42.00
226	Ester-C, 180 caplets, 550 mg. each	25.00
227	Flannel Cloth	5.00
228	Germanium, 200 mg., 30 tablets	45.00
229	Ginko-24, 60 mg., 60 tablets	25.00
312	Glutenzyme, 100 tablets, 330 mg each	16.00
230	Gold Stake, 60 capsules	30.00
285	Gold Stake, 125 capsules	58.00
232	Gozarte, 60 capsules	76.00
231	Gurmar, 90 capsules	19.00
233	Hepata-Quest (Liver), 90 capsules	16.00
200	HMF Forte, 45 capsules	25.00

Prod. No.	• *Healing Within Individual Items (cont.)*•	Price
286	Homozon, 150 grams	30.00
235	Immuno-Quest, 100 capsules	20.00
236	Infla-Zyme, 90 tablets	25.00
287	Infla-Zyme, 180 tablets	45.00
237	Intestinal Cleanser, Colon 8, 120 caplets	8.00
238	Intestinal Cleanser, Healing Within, 120 capsules	11.00
239	Intestinal Cleanser, Healing Within, 250 capsules	20.00
241	Intestinalis Herbal Cleanser, 60 tablets	29.00
288	Intracept, 60 tablets	25.00
242	K-Min, 180 capsules	14.00
243	Kapracidin-A, 90 capsules	$ 18.00
244	KB-11, 60 tablets	5.00
245	Latero Flora, 60 capsules	26.00
246	Lipoic Acid (thiotic)	24.00
320	Livit 2 Indian Herbal Food, 90 capsules, 500 mg. each	27.00
289	Maccalozon, 150 grams	30.00
290	Magdaclarin, 60 capsules	76.00
291	Magozone, 150 grms.	30.00
292	Melatone, 3 mgs./capsule, 60 capsules	20.00
251	Natur-Earth, 500 mg., 90 capsules (2 for $80.00)	42.50
253	Neo-Pararte, 60 capsules	76.00
255	Orithrush-D, 8 fl. oz. concentrate	14.00
293	OXY-MAG, 4 oz.	35.00
294	OXY-OXC, 180 capsules	30.00
256	Padapco, 60 capsules	76.00
295	Para-Citro, 60 capsules	76.00
257	Pasaloc, 60 capsules	76.00
258	Pau D'Arco Tea, 4 oz. bulk package	8.00
259	Pecta Sol, 450 grams, 16 oz. powder	165.00
262	Plus (Wild Mexican Yam DHEA), 90 capsules	39.00
260	Pro Sanoa (Saw Palmetto), 60 softgels, 160 mg. each	25.00
316	Prostex, 250 capsules	23.00
296	Pychogenol, 60 tablets	20.00
322	Replete, 7 sachets	30.00
297	Sanozone, 150 grms	30.00

Prod. No.	• *Healing Within Individual Items (cont.)*•	Price
298	Shark Cartilage, 750 mgs., 100 capsules	40.00
299	Shark Cartilage, 750 mgs., 300 capsules	99.00
263	Shitake Mushrooms, 90 capsules	20.00
264	Stinging Nettles, 90 capsules	20.00
265	Sub-Adrene, 15 ml., sub-lingual, dropper bottle	29.00
266	Sub-Germanium, 15 ml., sub-lingual, dropper bottle	29.00
267	Sub-Taurine, 1 oz., sub-lingual, dropper bottle	25.00
269	Travacid X, 100 caplets	18.00
324	Trifal, 90 capsules	23.00
270	Udarte, 60 capsules	76.00
271	Ultra Phos, 1 oz.	14.00
275	Vital Pak, 30 day supply	45.00
276	Vitamin E, Grace, 180 capsules	36.00
321	Poly VitaMyns Multi Vitamins & Minerals, 90 capsules	30.00
323	WheyPlex, 4 oz.	24.00
277	Whole Life Food Blend, 16 oz.	33.00
250	Mon Paradise, 500 mg., 60 capsules	$ 76.00
279	Pac-Pik, 500 mg., 60 capsules	76.00

Prod. No.	• **Books**•	Price
902	*Healing Within: The Complete Guide to Colon Health,* Stanley Weinberger	$ 15.95
906	*Parasites: An Epidemic in Disguise,* Stanley Weinberger	7.95
907	*Candida Albicans: The Quiet Epidemic,* Stanley Weinberger	11.95

Shipping & Product Information

Call or Fax Your Order: You may call or fax your order only with Visa, MasterCard, American Express, or Discover to *Healing Within Products.* Business hours are 8:00 a.m. to 5:00 p.m. Pacific Standard Time, Monday through Saturday.

Minimum Order: $25.00. Minimum Shipping Chg: $5.00.

Shipping Method: Orders are shipped via UPS Ground. For Second Day Blue Label delivery, double the shipping charges. No shipping on Saturdays, Sundays or legal holidays. Visa, MasterCard, American Express, and Discover orders are shipped on the next working day.

Alaska & Hawaii Shipments: For shipments to Alaska and Hawaii, double the continental U.S. shipping charge. Orders will be sent by U.S. First Class Mail.

Canada Shipments: For shipments to Canada, double the continental U.S. shipping charge. Orders will be sent by U.S. Air Parcel Post.

Overseas & Foreign Shipments: For overseas surface shipments, triple the shipping charge; allow 6 weeks for delivery. For overseas air orders, add five times the continental U.S. shipping charge. *All foreign accounts must send bank certified checks in U.S. dollars; credit cards accepted.*

Prices: Prices are subject to change without notice.

Returns: Any items you wish to return must have been purchased within the past 30 days. You cannot return opened bottles or bottles with defaced labels. All returns will have a 10% handling charge. All returned checks will be charged a $10.00 fee. If you are returning products by UPS, send to: *Healing Within Products,* 84 Berkeley Avenue, San Anselmo, CA 94960. If you are returning products by U.S. Postal Service, send to: *Healing Within Products,* P.O. Box 1013, Larkspur, CA 94977-1013

Product Storage: We suggest storing your supplements in a cool, dry location. The label will specify if refrigeration is required. These products are for nutritional supplementation only. They are not intended for the mitigation, cure or treatment of any disease or illness. No other use is assumed, implied, intended or permitted.

Healing Within Products

P.O. Box 1013 • Larkspur, CA 94977-1013 Orders Only (800) 300-7548 • in Calif. call (415) 454-6677 • Fax (415) 454-6659

Healing Within Products Order Form

Prod. No.	Product	Quantity	Price	Total

Minimum Order $25.00

Total Order

California residents add 7.5% tax

Each 4- to 7-Day Cleansing Kit Shipping, Handling & Insurance — $8.00
Each Three Phase Intestinal Flora Rebuilding Program Kit Shipping, Handling & Insurance — $10.00
Each Complete Parasite or Candida Elimination Kit Shipping, Handling & Insurance — $12.00

Shipping and Handling for individual items:
Minimum Shipping Charge $5.00. Up to $50 add 10% of individual item price; over $50 add 8%
(See detailed Shipping & Product Information)

TOTAL AMOUNT ENCLOSED

Fax and telephone orders accepted only with Visa, MasterCard, American Express, or Discovery. Credit card orders and orders paid with bank checks or money orders are shipped the next working day. Orders paid with personal check will be shipped in 10 days. Send personal check payable to *Healing Within Products*. No C.O.D. Prices subject to change.
Please print clearly:

Name _____ Day Phone (_____) _____

Address _____ Evening Phone (_____) _____

City _____ State _____ Zip _____

☐ Visa ☐ MasterCard ☐ Am. Ex. ☐ Discover   Card # _____

Expiration Date _____ Signature _____

OXYGEN
ACIDOPHILUS
NYSTATIN